CONFESSIONS, PERSPECTIVES, and REFLECTIONS OF A PARAMEDIC

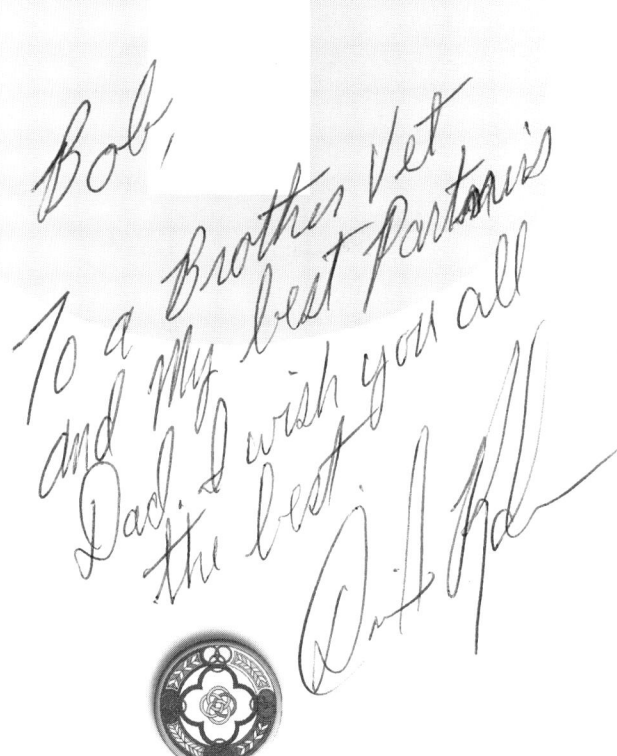

By David Ryden

TONE; Confessions, Perspectives, and Reflections of a Paramedic
Copyright © 2010 by David Ryden All rights reserved.

No part of this publication may be reproduced, stored in a retrieval system, or transmitted in any way by any means – electronic, mechanical, photocopy, recording, or otherwise – without the prior permissions of the copyright holder, except as provided by USA copyright law.

The information in this book is based on experiences of the author over a period of nearly four decades. Despite the authors desire to relate the many stories as accurately as possible, he will not be held responsible for the absolute certainty of all the information within this book. Since many of the stories and anecdotes are not verifiable with a 100% certainty, the author and the publisher will not be held responsible for any errors within the manuscript.

Published by: Brittane Publishing LLC
PO Box 10973 Bradenton, FL 34282
www.tonesbydavidryden.com

Book cover design and formatting: Eli Blyden
www.CrunchTimeGraphics.Net

ISBN 13: 978-0-578-08989-8

Biography/Autobiography/Memoir/Paramedic/Medical/EMS

Printed in the United States of America:
A&A Printing | www.printshopcentral.com

For James

IV TONES

Acknowledgements

This book would not have been possible without the help and encouragement of my friends Kevin Mills and Tony Klein, as well as my EMS brothers and sisters. I would also like to thank my family, especially my mom, for always being there for me.

VI TONES

CONTENTS

Dedications III
Acknowledgements V
Introduction 1
Chapter 1 7
Chapter 2 15
Chapter 3 21
Chapter 4 25
Chapter 5 35
Chapter 6 45
Chapter 7 49
Chapter 8 55
Chapter 9 59
Chapter 10 63
Chapter 11 71

VIII TONES

Chapter 12	87
Chapter 13	91
Chapter 14	97
Chapter 15	101
Chapter 16	107
Chapter 17	117
Chapter 18	123
Chapter 19	129
Chapter 20	137
Chapter 21	145
Chapter 22	149
Chapter 23	153
Chapter 24	163
Chapter 25	169
Chapter 26	179
Chapter 27	189
Chapter 28	193
Chapter 29	205
Chapter 30	213

INTRODUCTION

I am a paramedic, and have been for over 17 years. Kevin, my best friend since I was about two years old, has listened to me talk about my EMS (Emergency Medical Services) experiences, both good and bad, over the years, and he suggested that I write a book about them. He thought I should not only include just my EMS views, but also my opinions about life in general. At the very least, he thought that would make the book more entertaining.

  I explained to Kevin that I didn't know anything about writing a book. He suggested that I try to write down my thoughts just the same way I talk.

  When I mentioned Kevin's idea of writing a book to Tony, another one of my closest friends, he also thought it was something I should do. Tony and I became best friends while we served together in the Army, and he is the only person from my military days I still keep in touch with. After some prodding from my friends and thinking about it on and off for a while, I finally decided to give writing my story a try. So here it goes.

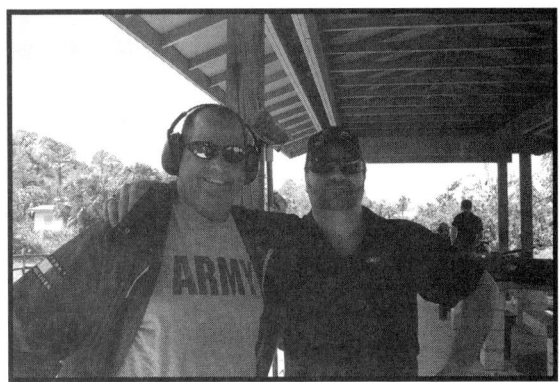
Me and my best friend since childhood Kevin, taking a break at the gun range.

Prior to becoming a paramedic, I was a soldier and served in the United States Army for six years. During this time I learned how to stand up for myself and speak my mind. Unfortunately, profanity is a big part of my vocabulary and for that I apologize. I call it like I see it and don't sugarcoat anything.

I've seen movies and TV shows that have EMS in their storylines. In my eyes they have all failed at capturing the true essence of the job and the people who work it. It seems like emergency workers are either portrayed as oversensitive drama types or burned-out losers. I would describe these portrayals as being too Hollywood, and by that I mean unrealistic. I'm not dogging the actors, but I am criticizing the people who have written the actors' words and storylines.

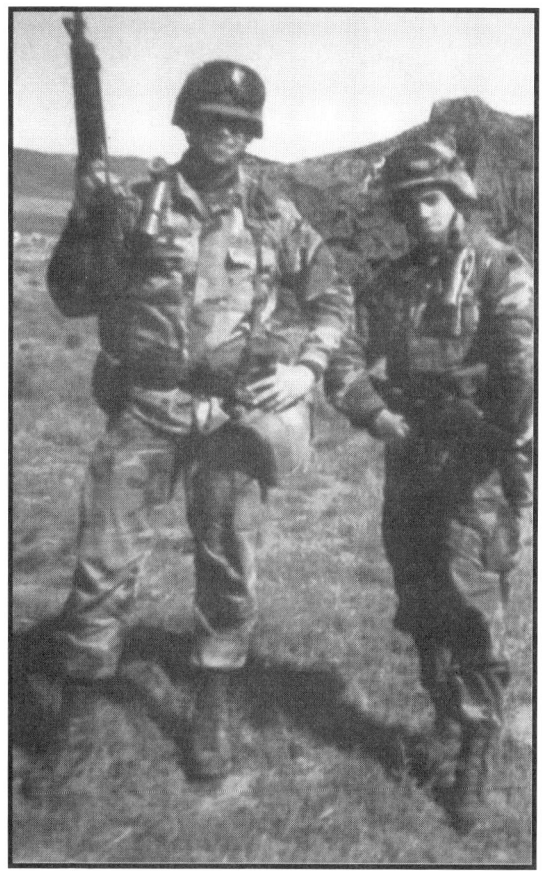

Me and Tony during our Army days.

The few books I've read on the subject have also fallen short of depicting EMS at its core. Hopefully I can paint a realistic picture of what it's like being in emergency workers' boots so you can get a true sense of what it's really like on the street as a medic. By no means am I trying to discourage people from getting into this field. I'm just trying to shine an honest light on this particular career.

You may have a friend or relative who works in EMS and totally disagrees with my views. That's all right. I can say, however, that everything you are about to read is true. The events and 911 calls mentioned in this book happened to me. At times I may stray into different health care topics, but in the end they relate to EMS.

I should also mention that in the emergency world other issues arise such as politics, religion, and other social topics so I'm not going to hold back when discussing these subjects either. I have seen and continue to see things that bother me. They just don't make any sense to me, so the fact that I'm finally putting pen to paper may help me figure them out. On these subjects you may agree with my views or think I'm a total ass. That's for you to decide.

I was raised in a conservative household, and in the past, I have always considered myself a Republican. As time has passed, however, I've observed the good and bad from both sides of the political spectrum, left and right. While I hate labels, I guess I'm now what may be considered an Independent, although I still lean right.

You know what, scratch that last sentence. I'm not an Independent either. I'm a realist, and unfortunately, folks like me don't have a party.

I'm sure that by the time you're done reading this book, I will have offended or pissed you off in some way. I assure you that that's not my intention, but it seems in this day and age, keeping everyone happy is impossible. I have developed a pretty thick skin over the years so I'm prepared for any negative feedback. Hopefully, whether you like this book or not, at the very least it will make you think. In the end, you may also learn a few things about the emergency world.

6 TONES

Chapter 1

I was born in California and raised in Florida. My father was a decorated war hero, and after his time in the military, he worked in the insurance industry. That's where he met my mom.

We moved to Florida when I was about two, and the town I grew up in didn't have much to offer kids, so most of us just hung out and got into trouble. Although my family has a long history of military service, I initially ignored it and spent my teen years as a slacker punk.

For a brief period I played sports and was actually one hell of a baseball player. I even attended a summer baseball camp put on by the Philadelphia Phillies where baseball greats like Larry Bowa and Mike Schmidt taught us the basics of the game. One year I was my team's MVP.

8 TONES

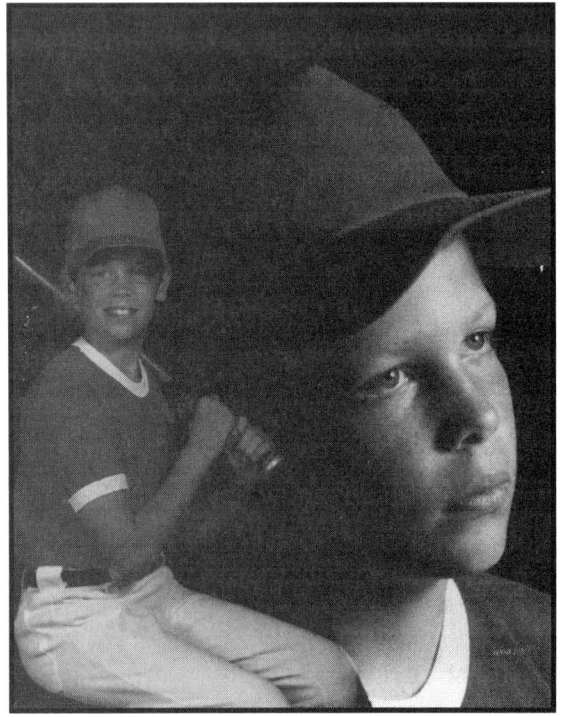

My baseball days.
I wish I still had that innocence in my eyes.

Unfortunately, sports got old for me and I hooked up with the wrong crowd. It was only after I realized I was going nowhere that I enlisted in the Army, which I knew I was destined to do anyway. There I found the direction I needed. Like my brief foray into sports, I was once again a member of a team, and I decided to make it a career.

I was stationed at Ft. Lewis in Washington after serving two year-long tours overseas. Out of all my time in the Army, it was only when I was serving out of country that I actually felt like a soldier. Ask any

Army veteran and they will tell you that stateside duty sucked, at least during the Cold War. Instead of looking across an expanse of land at an enemy who wants to kill you, in the states you practice walking in formation for some parade.

I can't even imagine what it must be like in today's Army, with all the hardships and combat tours these soldiers are seeing. But I wish I was still in.
I loved being a soldier but my father was sick with Parkinson's disease. My mom needed help back home in Florida taking care of him. My brother, Erik, was serving in the United States Air Force at that time, so I decided to leave the Army and return home to help Mom. When I decided to leave the Army, I was awaiting promotion to staff sergeant.

When I got back to Florida, I started looking for a job, but the big problem for me was the fact that all my real skills involved shooting things and blowing shit up. However, there was one thing I'd thought about doing for a long time, ever since I lived in Washington.

One time back then, I was at a girlfriend's apartment hanging out, when the TV show *Rescue 911* came on. The show basically recreated 911 calls and the episodes always seemed to have a happy ending involving the victim and his or her family having a picnic with the rescue workers. At the time, I thought that job was something I could do. I can also say, many years later, I'm still waiting for that first picnic.

On my return to Florida, I signed up at the local vocational school for the EMT/paramedic program. Prior to this I had only received very basic first aid training, and I wasn't quite sure what to expect. While I was in the Army, I went through a course called *combat lifesaver*, which taught a little bit more than boot camp, but it was nothing like what I was about to experience.

The first six months of learning for my new career was the EMT (Emergency Medical Technician) part of the program which taught basic first aid and how to assist a paramedic. The second portion, which lasted about a year, was the paramedic course.

Have you ever noticed how some people can pick up things such as math or sports naturally? Well, that is how para-medicine was for me. I wasn't book smart, and I totally sucked at studying for the exams, but I was able to quite easily pick up and retain the stuff I thought I would need as a street medic.

During both the EMT and paramedic courses, I did a lot of clinical ride time with the local EMS crews. That's where I *really* learned. Forget the classroom, put me on the street. Like the Army, I learned more *doing* than reading. I was very motivated and liked what I was learning. Emergency medicine fascinated me because I had no idea how much skill was involved.

Before EMS, the only true medically related emergencies I had encountered were when a fellow soldier in my unit was killed in a tank accident and another was wounded by a land mine. I was pretty naive as to what this emergency medical stuff was all about. The reality of it all came hard and fast on my first EMT clinical ride.

My very first call as a student involved an eight week old SIDS (Sudden Infant Death Syndrome) call. I was a new student, and the first time I did CPR (Cardio Pulmonary Resuscitation) on a real patient—not a dummy—was on a baby at a day care. I had no clue what the hell I was doing and I was scared shitless. The medic crew I was riding with, on the other hand, was calm, cool, and collected.

It was on this first call I learned that no matter what situation you find yourself in, you can't let it overwhelm you. Maintaining your composure is the key. People will feed off your reactions during a time of crisis.

Driving home from that first clinical ride, I wondered if I'd made the right decision or should I have stayed in the Army. Had I bitten off more than I could chew?

On my next clinical ride I had my first MVC (Motor Vehicle Crash) and it involved a fatality. A car was hit by a semi truck, and the young woman in the backseat was ejected through the rear window. She landed in the median partially under another car that had stopped. The driver of the stopped car freaked out and stepped on the gas, squashing the ejected girl's head.

On my first clinical I had seen a dead baby, and on this one, only my second ride, I saw a person's brains splattered across a highway. It didn't faze me. I knew right then I had the stomach to do this job. I had made the right decision.

In the paramedic program a student is taught ALS (Advanced Life Support) skills. You learn how to start IV's, perform endotracheal intubations, manually defibrillate, administer medications, assist in delivering babies, perform needle and surgical cricothyrotomies and chest decompressions, and a lot of other stuff. You may not understand the words or procedures I just mentioned, so even though I hate the show, watch a couple episodes of *ER*. It may help you understand what I am talking about.

Toward the end of paramedic school, I applied with my county's EMS service. Even though there was a long waiting list, I got hired. I couldn't believe it. There were a lot more experienced people than me who had applied, but I got the job.

It would be a year or so later before I found out why. It turned out the female training captain who did my interview had also been one of my paramedic instructors, and she was attracted to me, which she confided to me later. I still find that hard to believe. It was kind of funny because as a student I had always wanted to ask her out but I didn't have the guts. We actually dated for a while, but like all of my other relationships, I screwed it up ... but that's another story.

Anyway, I got the job I had been training for, so I'm not complaining.

After two years of living on the GI Bill, it was awesome to finally be earning what I thought at the time was a decent paycheck. It didn't take long for me to learn that the EMS service I worked for paid a lot less than most services in my area.

My schedule was, and still is, 24 hours on, and 48 hours off. It would seem to some that this schedule is like getting a weekend off after every day of work. The only problem is, if you have a shift where you run your ass off for 24 hours straight, your first day off is pretty much wasted. You are mentally and physically drained, and it takes half a day to re-energize.

After all these years I wouldn't know how to work a 9 to 5 job because I never have. My first job was a dish pig (dishwasher) when I was 13 or 14, and those hours varied. I've been working ever since, and over the last 17 years my body and mind have adjusted to the 24-hour shift.

14 TONES

CHAPTER 2

My first partner was a guy named Butch, who I consider the best medic that ever walked the earth. Today he works as a physician's assistant at a couple of the local hospitals.

Butch taught me so much; the main thing he taught me was to use common sense. You'll find as you read this book, I have zero tolerance for people without common sense.

I always told myself that if I could be one-tenth the medic that Butch was, I'd be a good one. I think I've achieved that. The trick is—you need fifty percent experience and the other fifty percent common sense.

This job, contrary to what some people in my field might have you believe, is not rocket science. One of my co-workers said it best, "Our classroom was right next to the classroom where the people learned how to fix boat motors." It doesn't take a genius, just the right mentality.

The service I work for is its own entity. We are not part of a fire department but strictly EMS, and we run about 40,000 calls a year. It seems to me that most people have the misconception that all paramedics and ambulances are part of the fire service. The fact is, there are many EMS services nationwide, both government and private, not associated with a fire department.

I read about a study in one of the emergency magazines lying around the station. It found that *stand alone* EMS departments actually give better medical care than departments that provide both fire and EMS service. The study concluded that you can either be an outstanding firefighter or an outstanding paramedic, but you may sometimes be subpar if expected to do both.

For my fire medic friends, I'm sorry, and I do realize it's just one study. Granted, there are many exceptions to the rule. I know medics who started in my service before leaving for a fire department, and they are outstanding medics. I think the primary reason they're outstanding is because they started out in an EMS-only service.

Those who have the power to increase our pay use the excuse that since people like me are only paramedics and not also firefighters, our low pay is justified. That's total BS. The firefighter/paramedics in the adjoining areas run medical calls just like me, and are rarely, if ever, called upon to fight fires. I have a lot of friends who are firefighters, and I will never disrespect them or the fire service. They are brave, they are heroes, and I won't take that away.

The public's idea of the emergency services as a whole is distorted and messed up. A few years ago my partner and I were at an Arby's restaurant getting lunch. Despite the fact that two stores from this chain have disrespected me while I was on duty, I love their roast beef sandwich. Anyway, I was at the counter with people behind me when the young girl behind the register called her manager over and asked for a key so she could give me a discount.

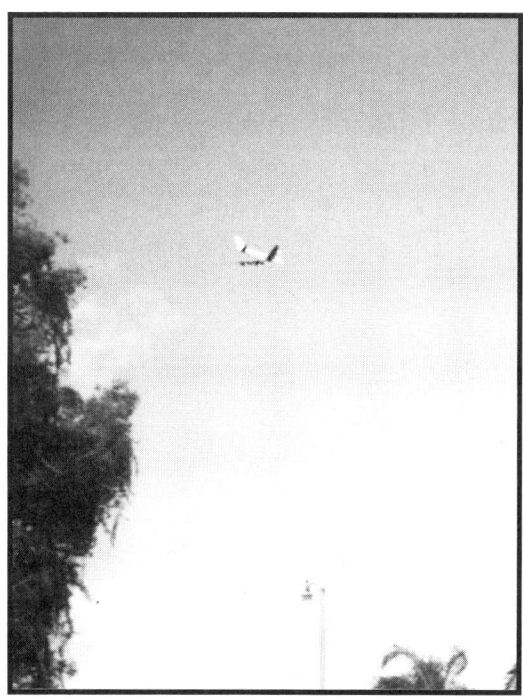

Air force one flying over my station
shortly after the 9/11 attacks.

Some places will give us a discount. We never ask but it is appreciated. The manager looked at me, and in front of all my fellow customers said, "He's only EMS. We don't give discounts to them, just fire and police."

I could tell the cashier was very embarrassed for me, and I told her not to sweat it because I get disrespected every day. I wished I could have explained to all of them the reality of emergency work. With today's fire suppression systems and alarms, everyone will be outside before a fire engulfs the building. If you are robbed and shot, though, don't expect the cops to be there until after the fact—unless by some freak chance some cop is in the drive-through getting a roast beef supreme.

The truth is, the people whose asses they should be kissing are the EMS workers. While you are bleeding to death, the cops will be putting up crime tape and yelling at me for tramping through their scene. The firefighters will be assisting me, while I am using all of my advanced skills trying to save you.

Who's worth the discount now? Like I said, discount or not, myself and people like me are your first shot at survival. The public have had a distorted view of EMS for a long time. It's a shame but it *is* reality.

Just look at America's reaction to the events of September 11, 2001. I was actually working the day of the 9-11 attacks and have a photo I took of Air Force One as it flew over my station. My partner, Jackie, and

I watched the Twin Towers fall on TV, as did most of the nation.

As an Army veteran who had spent time defending this country, it all made me sick. Thousands of innocent civilians died, as well as firefighters, police, and yes, EMS workers.

In the days that followed, you didn't hear much about the medics who died. I saw a few tributes that briefly mentioned EMS, and I thought that was nice. But as is the norm, it was mostly fire and police.

I personally didn't know anyone who perished, and my thoughts and prayers have always gone out to their families. Since the tragedy, the emergency world I live in feels a need to celebrate on 9-11. In my town they have various events, and a party at the convention center. Some of the local fire, police, and I'm sorry to say, EMS workers, get shitfaced and pose like heroes.

Not unlike December 7, I believe September 11 should be a day of remembrance, not celebration. I'm sure those families affected aren't celebrating.

Someone once asked me if I was going to participate in any of the 9-11 festivities, and I said, "Hell no! If people who don't appreciate my service 364 days out of the year want to call me a hero for one day to make themselves feel good, they can kiss my ass. I would have more respect for them if they would just treat me like dirt for 365 days."

I have integrity, another thing I learned in the Army. I really can't stand *brownnosers*, which unfortunately describes some people in the emergency field. I won't take any credit for something I wasn't a part of.

I'm not saying that the entire public treats us badly, and in all honesty, I believe the majority are very thankful. It's just that most people have no clue what calling an ambulance is all about. The fact that they are getting what amounts to a mobile emergency room with highly skilled medical professionals showing up at their door seems to escape them.

Writing my thoughts down is a new experience for me, and I'm learning as I go, but I thought some background was needed. As a new member of the EMS team, I was all about serving the community. Saving lives and easing suffering was the job, or so I thought. When the tones (annoying, sustained, blaring noises sent out over a loudspeaker) went off, alerting us to a call, I would jump up, and rush to the unit/truck (ambulance).

It didn't take long for me to realize that most of the calls we got were bullshit. I mean, why the hell am I going, lights and sirens, to foot pain? Unless the foot has been traumatically amputated, there is nothing life-threatening about *that*.

The powers that be, however, think differently. *The people calling might sue if we don't get there quickly*—that's *their* train of thought. I guess potentially causing vehicle accidents with bystanders being injured by traffic stopping quickly for my *Mobile Electric Light Orchestra* is acceptable to them.

Chapter 3

A brief view of the service and the area I work in. We cover everything from the beach to the rural farmland. Besides the service I work for, there are roughly ten separate fire departments in my county. Both the fire departments and EMS have three, 24-hour shifts—A, B, and C.

Over the years I have worked on every shift and have run calls with almost every firefighter in town. We all work as a team, and most of our EMS units are stationed at various firehouses. I am assigned to one of our few stations not located at a firehouse. My station is an old double wide trailer, nothing fancy, but we call it home away from home.

Some firefighters look at our emergency crews as if we are an annoyance or we're invading their space. The firefighters that I work with on my shift, B shift, and the ones in my zone, are awesome. I must admit that there is some friction that goes on in some fire stations which is caused by the EMS crews. Some kids just don't play well with others.

The local firefighters and police in my town are paid substantially more than the EMS workers, even if they have less time served and run significantly fewer calls. Some firefighters make a point of reminding us about that fact and that's a shame. Remember Arby`s?

Speaking of running calls, I would have to say, and many of my co-workers agree, that roughly 75 percent of the calls we run are not even close to real emergencies. Before I start giving examples, which by the way is my main purpose for writing, I must offer this piece of advice. If you have a loved one who suffers or dies because of a delay in ALS (Advance Life Support) care arriving promptly, research it. Chances are the closest ambulance was on a bullshit call and couldn't assist you because of repercussions that would befall the medic crew if they left the bullshit to come to your aid. Trust me, we want to help you, but our hands are tied.

When I started, I didn't care what kind of call it was. Lighting up the roof and spinning the siren used to make me feel important. The way traffic got out of the way kind of made me feel like Moses parting the Red Sea, although Moses didn`t have to deal with Q-tips (old folks), or people blabbing or texting on cell phones slowing down the sea. He didn't have to deal with the drunk passed out by the dumpster, the old man stuck on a toilet, or some shoplifter faking a seizure.

Anyway, none of it got me down at first. I was there to run calls, and save the world. *Bring it on,* I thought. What a dumbass I was! If I could go back in time, I would kick my own ass. I think all of us in EMS start out the same. We just want to help people and try to make a difference. On rare occasions we actually do.

I remember my first *code* or *Cardiac Arrest* save. This old guy coded on a golf course, and my partner and I busted our asses working on him. We were able to get a pulse back en route to the hospital, and a few weeks later we got a rare thank you letter from his wife. She said he recovered and was at home. I felt really good about that, because had it not been for our actions, he wouldn't have survived.

Unfortunately, calls like that are few and far between. Since then I have been involved with close to 100 code saves, most of which were brain dead even though we got the heart started. Don't get me wrong, it has and always will feel good when you can get off shift knowing that you made a positive impact on someone's life. It's just that a lot of times, no matter how hard you try, regardless of the type of call, to some people it's never good enough. In this line of work you see both the best and worst of society. You just have to gear yourself to deal with people and situations one call at a time.

24 TONES

Chapter 4

Let's say you are a medic. Your shift begins at 7 a.m. and you spend the first 10 or 15 minutes bullshitting with the off-going crew. They let you know if there is anything that might need special attention on the unit and describe any interesting calls they may have encountered.

Examples of an interesting call could include something like a really bad MVC (Motor Vehicle Collision), a code, or some idiot who called for something so dumb it boggles the mind. After crew change, you check out your truck. You inspect your medications for accountability and expiration dates. O2 (Oxygen) levels are checked and you go through the kits. These include your medical/IV kit, oxygen bag, and heart monitor. In my service there are also kits specifically for trauma and pediatrics.

When you're done with the unit checkout, you sit back and wait for the games to begin. The tones can go off at any time. Sometimes you don't get the first call for hours, and other times you get it right when you walk through the door.

I personally show up to work with the expectation of going straight from my car to the unit for a call. In the zone (assigned area) I work, an average 24-hour shift consists of approximately 8 to 14 calls. This varies depending on the time of year. In the winter months we run more calls because of all the *snow birds*, another term for old people who come down from the north.

The snowbird migration to Florida is something like the wildebeest migration in Africa that Butch told me about when I started working with him. The old and weak make the trek with the rest of the herd and then become ill or die upon reaching their destination. It must be awesome working EMS in Michigan during the winter months.

After the tones alert you to a call, they are followed by a 911 dispatcher's voice giving you information about the type of call and the address. Dispatchers, whether you love them or hate them, are your lifeline. Sometimes it feels as if they are creating calls just to keep you running. It's easy to blame them, but down inside you know they're just doing a job. If you're on a call and realize you need extra hands such as the fire department to help lift a large patient, dispatch sends them. If you're on a call and some dickbag decides he wants to go UFC (Ultimate

Fighting Champion) on your ass, dispatch is your only hope. You actually have emergency buttons on your portable radios if you find yourselves in a world of hurt and need help.

I know it's hard to believe, but not everyone will welcome you with open arms. There are a lot of crazy bastards out there who hate your ass even though they called you for help. Needless to say, my compassion levels plummet when dealing with these buttwads.

It`s 9 a.m. and the first call comes in. "Chest pain," dispatch advises, and within 30 seconds you're en route to the call. A computer in the truck gives you the call location on a map and additional information about the call. A 97 year old female at a nursing home is having chest pain and shortness of breath. Five minutes after being toned out, you're on scene.

The staff members working at the home look at you with clueless, blank expressions. It takes three minutes to find someone who supposedly knows what the hell is going on. You're given paperwork with patient info and led to the room. You're told the patient has been having chest pain since breakfast. Entering the room, you find the patient motionless in bed. Maybe you're too late. Nope, she is just sleeping. After you almost literally scare her to death by waking her up, you start asking her questions. Quickly realizing she's deaf as a doornail, you soon find yourself shouting in her ear.

The patient is clearly in no distress, so you turn to ask the staff member why you were called. Unfortunately, she has already left the room. Leaving your partner with the non-patient, you begin your hunt for the so-called nurse who brought you to the room. One of the kitchen staff employees says he saw her enter a break room, and it is there you find your prey feeding her face, and yakking on a cell phone.

Inquiring as to why exactly you were called, she informs you that after breakfast the old lady burped and touched her chest. The lady's doctor was called prior to your arrival and has given orders that she be transported to the hospital for evaluation. Even though you know there is absolutely nothing wrong with her, you are in no position to argue the *common sense* of letting her go back to sleep. Trust me, in this job arguing common sense is a losing battle. You simply load her up and haul her away, or as we sometimes call it, *Sling a Lizard.* It's a term I didn't create, and I can only assume it comes from the fact that the elderly in Florida often have sun-baked, wrinkled skin.

Maybe now you get some idea as to why Medicare is so messed up. Heaven forbid the lowly paramedic say anything!

After arriving at one of the local emergency rooms, you have to explain to the nursing staff what is wrong with the patient. The majority of nurses you deal with are awesome, and some of these girls are smoking hot. I should mention that there are male nurses also, but no need to dwell on that. There are some nurses, however, who are total assholes regardless of gender and they look at you with disdain. I think some actually think you drive around looking for patients to bring them. Trust me, I'd much rather be sitting on my butt back at the station playing video games.

Nurses, good or bad, are the ones who run the ER. Yes, there are doctors, but they would be lost if not for the nursing staff. Anyway, you explain the old lady's situation. After the nurses shake their heads just like you did back at the nursing home, they take her off your hands. First call down.

It's 9:45 a.m. and you return to the station. Just as you get back in zone you receive the next call. As soon as you hear the address, you feel like your head is going to explode. Dispatch simply advises the call type as *Sick Person*, but you and your partner know exactly what kind of call this is going to be. The so-called *sick person* is actually a worthless, drunken piece of shit you run into on almost every shift.

Frequent Flyer is the term you use to describe people like this. "I wish this sorry, worthless waste of space, would just die already!" you tell your partner while en route.

Upon arrival you find this upstanding member of society standing in the front yard of a rundown house wearing only his tighty-whities and shitting all over himself. "Don't ask any questions, and just take me to the fucking hospital!" he demands.

It takes all of your restraint to refrain from beating the living shit out of him. Once again, you must grin and bear it, knowing your unit may be unable to respond to a real emergency due to this guy.

The smell from this a guy is so foul, your partner and you have to put face masks on so as not to puke during transport. Upon arrival at the ER, you find out the nurse you're getting is one of the bad ones, a real bitch, and with that you get a sense of satisfaction knowing you just ruined her day with your latest delivery. *Sometimes Karma is a wonderful thing.* While you are transferring patient care to the nurse, your partner has the back of the unit opened up and is working feverishly to remove the drunken shit stench.

As you're walking out to the truck, another crew arrives with a crazed-looking drug addict who is restrained to the stretcher, who looks to be trying to eat his own face. "That's a shame," you say to the crew with a smile. "Screw you!" is the reply.

Oh, what brotherly love! These people you work with are your brothers and sisters. Like any family, though, there are some members you get along with better than others, but you would do *anything* for any of them.

With the unit now *defunked*, you return to the station. The rest of the morning is uneventful. Noon comes and you and your partner decide to go to a local hole in the wall diner for lunch.

You hate eating out when on duty because somebody always wants to interrupt and ask you for medical advice—like you can pretend to give a shit about some old guy's hemorrhoids while you're trying to eat. Sometimes, though, the food is worth it, and working the streets, you learn all the best places in town to eat. If you ever find yourself in a new town and want to find a good place to eat, just ask an ambulance crew.

Just as the food arrives, the next call comes in. It's Murphy's Law. It's an MVC, and as you respond, dispatch advises they are receiving multiple 911 calls about it. That's never a good sign.

Upon arrival, you see an overturned SUV, and the fire crew that arrived shortly before you is doing CPR on a female lying in the road. *Walking* up to the patient, you never run, you realize there is nothing you can do. She has obviously received injuries that are not compatible with life.

Not to sound insensitive, but she is DRT (dead right there*)* or ART (assuming room temperature) or FUBAR (fucked up beyond all repair). These descriptions are crude, but you learned a long time ago that if you don't have a sense of humor in this job, you won't make it.

You instruct the firefighters to cease resuscitation efforts. On a medically-related scene the paramedics are in charge. Pronouncing a person dead is something you never get used to, but some people are beyond help. In this case the woman has an open skull fracture with brain matter protruding from it.

A crowd of bystanders has gathered on the side of the road. Some are crying while others are taking pictures with their cell phones. At least one is screaming at you for not doing anything.

Ignoring these idiots, you focus on the scene. This was a single vehicle accident, and you try to figure out what happened. It doesn't take long. The dead woman, probably in her thirties, sometimes it's hard to tell, is still clinching her cell phone in a partially amputated hand. This pisses you off because you know that, if she had been wearing a seat belt and paying attention to the road, she would still be alive. She crossed lanes on a curve and overcorrected, flipping her vehicle. Now all you can do is put a sheet over her. Oh well, back to lunch.

Throughout the rest of the day, you run a handful of calls, none being noteworthy. It's 10 p.m. and your last call was two hours ago. You and your partner make your bunks and lay down, hoping for a night's sleep.

No such luck. The tones blast you out of bed at 1 a.m. I'm not sure why, but it seems like the dumbest people on the planet come out of the woodwork after midnight. This call is no exception. Law enforcement's on the scene with some genius who decided to huff spray paint and then fell through a sliding glass door. You find this asshole sliced up from head to toe, and he's so high, he's laughing about it. Trying not to get blood all over ourselves, your partner and you bandage him up and take him to the hospital. It's a shame stupidity isn't always fatal.

It takes about an hour to clean off all the blood from the stretcher and the back of the unit. Just as you get back to the station, the tones go off again.

You ask yourself, *How is this possible? What gods did we piss off?* It's as if people wait for you to get back in zone before they call 911. We were gone for two hours, and now suddenly there's an emergency. This ends up being your last call of the shift, and it's for the same old lady you started out with.

Once again, she is sleeping, only this time permanently. Nature has taken its course. Good for her. Now these idiots won't be waking her up anymore. The shift ends and you've accomplished your main goal. Your partner and you made it out alive.

34 TONES

CHAPTER 5

Now that I have put you through a typical work day in my world, I feel that I should go into further detail about some of the stuff I just mentioned. Medicare and health insurance are totally abused in my opinion. Nursing homes calling for stupid and meaningless bullshit are just the tip of the iceberg. There is so much abuse going on that it would make any rational person sick, because in the long run, all of us hardworking tax payers are paying for it.

Some medical clinics are associated with certain hospitals. A patient will go to the clinic for a routine checkup, and the clinic will call 911 because their evaluation of the patient turned up something they say requires an ambulance transport to … *guess where*? To the hospital the clinic is affiliated with, of course.

I've actually argued with some of the staffs at clinics because the patient wants to go to a non-affiliated hospital. I must admit, sometimes I recommend another hospital to the patient solely to piss off the staff.

On many occasions I have transported patients like these, and upon my evaluation, I've found nothing out of the ordinary. The clinic would disagree, and I suppose I would too if I had what amounts to two paychecks riding on this one patient.

You see, if an ambulance is utilized to transport a patient, most insurance companies will pay because they believe it was medically warranted, even if there was nothing wrong with the patient. I don't have any proof, but it is my belief that the clinics, in turn, will be compensated for the clinic visit *and* by the receiving hospital. Certain wallets get fatter while the rest of us pay the tab with increased taxes.

Do I say anything about it? Not if I want to keep my job. In modern society, doctors are looked at as *gods* and their words as gospel. In my eyes, someone running bogus calls like these are no different than the asshole huffing paint. They're preventing me from caring for the truly sick and injured.

From what I've heard, emergency services aren't innocent either. I've heard some medics say they've discovered that PCR's (Patient Care Reports) they've turned in have been changed without their knowledge. Even if the report stated the call was not medically warranted, it was altered to reflect that it was. If this is true, then insurance companies and Medicare are paying out for people who did not deserve it. This, in turn, depletes Medicare and causes health insurance rates to skyrocket.

My department even had a guy from the billing service in Miami come and talk to us. He suggested ways we could write our reports so insurance companies would pay, even if the patient wasn't having any legitimate problem. I couldn't believe my ears. This guy was trying to get us to be part of the national health care problem.

I must clarify that the doctors I bring patients to in the emergency rooms are truly concerned about the patients' welfare. It's just a messed up system. Ambulance chasing lawyers and the fake claim-making clients that they represent are another huge burden on EMS and society in general.

Welfare is a friggin joke! I can't tell you how many times I've run calls on people because they wanted what amounts to a free ride to the hospital so they can get what amounts to free treatment because they're on welfare. Some of these same people have brand new cars in their driveways and satellite dishes on their roofs. I've actually stood behind people like this at the grocery store and watched as they buy a hundred dollars worth of booze and cigarettes, and then they pull out food stamps for cheese. Even worse, some of them aren't even legal residents. What the hell? The political correctness in this country has gone too far.

If some people want to donate their money to these so-called unfortunates, that is their right, but stop taking my hard earned money when I see firsthand how it is being wasted. I will gladly give donations to those who are legitimately mentally or physically disabled. As a matter of fact, I already do. I have supported the Special Olympics for years, as well as the United Service Organization and the Wounded Warrior Project, and have thank you cards to prove it. I'm just sick and tired of seeing hardworking people's money given to lazy people bucking the system.

What I'm about to mention will either shock some folks or piss them off, and I guess that's the point. One time we were sent to an assault call in an apartment complex. We showed up at the address that was given to law enforcement and knocked on the door. The door flew open and a girl in her twenties started cursing us out.

"Get the fuck out of here, assholes!" she shouted.

"Ma'am, did you call 911?" I asked.

"Do I look like I called 911? Get your asses out of my face!" She slammed the door as we backed off.

Obviously she had not called, and as we walked away, I noticed the door hadn't closed all the way. I could hear the woman talking to someone inside. She said, "The only time I want to see government people is when they cash my welfare check."

This would be the same girl begging me for help a couple days later after her man kicked the shit out of her. The hell with her, and the bleeding heart mentality that's infecting this country. I guess expecting her to go out and get a job instead of cranking out babies like it's a hobby is too much to ask in modern society. I'm sure you've heard the term "Babies Daddy". This refers to the biological father of a child not married to the mother. Some women will have multiple babies from different fathers, and collect separate welfare benefits for each. I have been on calls where I've heard people joking about having another child so they could afford to buy a flat screen TV.

Even worse, the majority of these *system abusers* I run on aren't having anything closely resembling a true medical emergency. Once again, while I'm tied up with them, you die.

Ask the rich politicians and celebrities about their high class medical insurance policies. Let me stop and clarify something before I go any further as I don't want to corral every celebrity into a certain group. There are many celebrities from every art form and political point of view who support and give generously to various charitable causes, and they should be applauded. I'm talking about the clueless ones who have no grasp on reality and still run their mouths. Because they have access to national media, they broadcast their ignorant and unrealistic views on health care across the country, and sadly, some people buy into it.

As far as medical insurance goes, I'm sure they'll either say it was included in some contract or they have an assistant to handle such trivial stuff. They won't get special treatment from me, I guarantee it. In a way, I look forward to the day I have one of them in the back of my truck, even if it's solely to educate them on the reality of the world I live in.

Trust me, I will give them the best care I possibly can, while letting them know they aren't special. After all, that's how the system has treated EMS workers and a lot of other hardworking folks busting their asses trying to make ends meet. I am an equal opportunity hater. If someone is a lazy, worthless piece of shit that milks the government tit and lives off my hard-earned money, I don't care what color or religion they are. In my eyes they deserve an ass beating.

Of course, you would have to work down at the level of an EMS professional (in the gutter) to appreciate that. Does this sound harsh? I sure as hell hope so. Because until right now, I have yet to see anyone remotely attempt to find justice or fairness for people, men and women alike, in my career field. So please, let me be the first to tell it like it is.

How is it possible that some people in the so-called entertainment industry and politicians are treated as if they are mythological gods? Am I missing something? Have I just awoken from a deep sleep? Don't get me wrong, I love movies and music, but I don't think these people are any better than the down-on-their-luck, homeless person who lost everything because of someone else's greed or incompetence. As for politicians, although they don't increased ticket prices, let's be honest, they all suck and they all lie regardless of party affiliations. When did the priorities of this world get so twisted? Maybe it was in my pre-army days when I was a slacker. I guess I'll never know.

Picture this, it's Thanksgiving Day, and you are sitting down to a beautiful dinner with the family. Grandma and Grandpa are there, as well as the kids and grandkids, and the smell of turkey and cranberries fills the air. Your Uncle Joe, who you haven't seen in years, has even made a surprise visit. A crisp fall breeze blows outside as the family gathers for a wonderful feast.

Suddenly, Grandpa clutches his chest, and is so short of breath he can't speak. While the rest of the family panics, the oldest grandson calls 911, which he was taught by trade school educated EMS workers during a visit to his school.

There is soon a knock at the door, and when it is opened, you see two figures standing at the threshold. On the left is a handsomely dressed, mega-rich politician, and on the right is a weary-looking paramedic with his kits in hand. It's your choice. Who do you want treating Grandpa, and who's worth the mighty dollar now?

I can tell you that, without any hesitation or reservation, the medic would be at Grandpa's side rendering aid regardless of being paid. It's in our nature, the same as it is for bureaucrats to downplay the importance of our profession.

It's like the old tale of the frog and the scorpion. The scorpion asks the frog to give him a lift across a stream. "Why should I do that?" the frog replies. "You'll just sting me, and I'll die." After a brief pause, the scorpion answers, "Why would I do that? If I sting you crossing the stream, we'll both die." After thinking it over the frog agrees, and the scorpion climbs on his back. Halfway across the stream, the scorpion stings the frog. "Why would you do that?" asks the frog. "Now we'll both die." As they start to sink, the scorpion replies, "I can't help it. It's in my nature."

I have a feeling that if I'm reincarnated, I'll come back as a frog. You see, just as it is in some people's nature to inflict pain and suffering on others without remorse, it is in an EMS worker's nature to render aid.

My opinion may be prejudiced due to the job, but it is my belief that paramedics, by nature, care more about the patient than anyone involved in their treatment. The only exception may be some of the nurses who also develop bonds. Nurses, however, are usually assigned multiple patients to keep track of, whereas an EMS crew deals with them one at a time and is with them from the beginning of their emergency.

I should clarify that by *patient* I mean an individual with a real need of medical attention, not just anyone who calls an ambulance, as I've already mentioned. Be it an AMI (Acute Myocardial Infarction), commonly known as a heart attack, a MVC (Motor Vehicle Crash), or a broken hip, EMS personnel are with the patient from the beginning. Many times we develop a bond with the patient. They're scared and look to us for comfort and reassurance. Although we never want to lie to a patient, sometimes we find ourselves doing it anyway.

44   TONES

CHAPTER 6

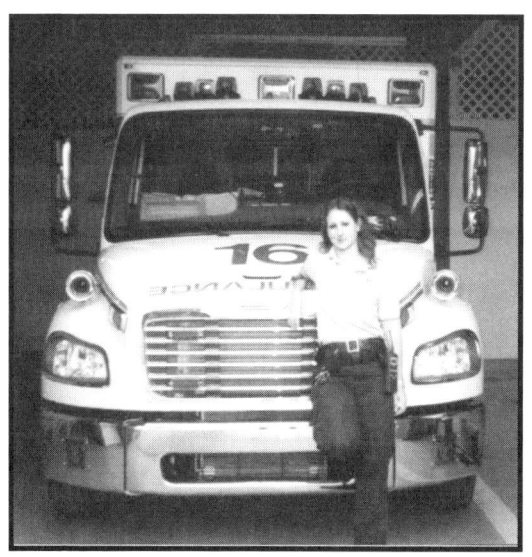

Angie chilling out between calls.

Words can't really describe the helpless feeling of trying to save a person you know is going to die. My newest partner, Angie, and I recently had a shooting victim who fell into this category. He was 30 years old and it was a drug deal that went bad. This guy had been shot with an assault rifle half a dozen times with entrance and exit wounds to his back and chest.

In my eyes he was already dead, he just didn't know it. He was begging me to save his life. I told him that he wasn't going to die—which in the EMS world is a cardinal sin—and we were doing everything we could for him. Moments after I intubated him (placed a flexible plastic tube into his trachea), he went into cardiac arrest.

Now this guy was a gangbanger with a long criminal record so I didn't really care about his outcome, but I was pissed at myself because I had lied to him. I should have just said "Hey dude, you wanted to live the thug life, now you get the thug death."

Over the years I have seen my share of patients die and I never get used to it. I've heard their last words and witnessed last breaths as the pupils dilate and fix.

"I think I'm about to die," "Tell my kids I love them," or "Please don't let me die." I think I've heard them all. Knowing that I have been the last person someone sees as their life fades away is hard to describe, so I won't even try.

I do believe in God and a life after this one, but that doesn't make it any easier. It's hard to remember my perception of life prior to EMS. I didn't know the finality of it, and the fact that when your time's up, it's up. Unlike the movies, there is nothing romantic or glamorous about death. I had a patient who smoked two packs a day and drank beer like a fish, and he lived to be a hundred. Another patient worked out daily, yet he dropped dead at the age of 40. There's neither rhyme nor reason.

When you aren't accustomed to death, I think life is more enjoyable. Hauling ass on a crotch rocket is a lot more fun when you haven't seen a human body torn apart after crashing one. Life and death is still a mystery to me.

Speaking of death, it amazes me how some people react when confronted with it. I remember a call where a woman met us in front of a condo wearing only a towel. "You people need to hurry the hell up!" she screamed. After a while you learn how to tune out people like this. The patient is the main concern, not some hysterical idiot. We found a male in his fifties, naked in bed, wearing a condom, with a bottle of Viagra on the nightstand. The patient was in cardiac arrest so we moved him to the floor and started working on him.

After defibrillating (shocking) his heart, I prepared my airway equipment for intubation. As I slid the endotracheal tube through his vocal cords, I couldn't help but hear the now calm woman talking on the phone. "You're not getting a dime! He cared about me more than you," she said into the phone. "You and your so-called lawyer can talk to these assholes who are working on him. He dropped dead while he was fucking me!"

I couldn't believe what I was hearing. Granted, this guy died the ultimate death in any man's eyes, but he wasn't even cold yet and this money-grubbing lady already had him buried. Now that's true love.

Chapter 7

Like the *towel lady*, money is on a lot of people's minds, including mine. I guess one of my main complaints is how shitty EMS workers are paid. I am on my eighteenth year as a paramedic for the same service, and I don't even make 15 dollars an hour, whereas a nurse *fresh out of school* starts at around 30 dollars an hour at a local ER. If you don't know the difference between a registered nurse and a paramedic, let me break it down.

While in school, both study anatomy, physiology, pharmacology, and various hands-on skills. Nursing, being a degree, also requires elective classes. At the end, nurses are licensed and medics are certified. This, I have been told, is why there is such a large pay difference.

Other than the words *registered* and *certified*, there are few differences between medics and nurses. In fact many hospital emergency rooms around the country are hiring medics because, as is the national standard, they're paid less than nurses and can actually do more. Although medics spend less time in school than nurses, paramedics are trained to deal with a larger assortment of medical issues than nurses.

In my career I have helped deliver babies and diagnosed and treated AMI's. I've performed critical surgical procedures such as cricothyrotomies and chest decompressions in the field, which is something nurses can't do. I have resuscitated countless numbers of patients from cardiac arrest.

I know I mentioned before that most code saves are brain dead, but I've had about 20 make it home. That's 20 people I have brought back from clinical death so they could die another day.

What makes my pay rate even worse is that there are medics in the surrounding counties who make substantially more than my co-workers and me. The medics in one of our adjoining counties make twice as much as us and also have two paid days off a month. Why don't I go work for another county? The way I look at it, I would rather stay and try to make justifiable changes here, where my friends and my family live.

All of the aforementioned *heroics*, like code saves, came without a doctor present. (I'm just joking about the hero thing.) Nurses work under the supervision of a physician and must have their orders before they can administer any treatment. Most of the nurses I know shouldn't have to wait for orders because they already know what the patient needs and what orders will be given.

I can't say enough about the ER nurses I deal with. They are awesome but there are enough books and TV shows about nurses and doctors, and this is *my* story. Paramedics, on the other hand, work under protocols that are set forth by each EMS Services' Medical Director. Usually these are doctors who work in one of the local emergency rooms. Following the set protocols, a medic doesn't need a doctor on scene giving orders to administer care. We evaluate the patient and determine what we believe will be the best course of action.

All paramedics are certified in ACLS (Advanced Cardiac Life Support), ITLS (International Trauma Life Support), and are held to the same standards as doctors in these subjects. My department, like many departments, also requires us to be certified in either PALS (Pediatric Advanced Life Support) or PEPP (Pediatric Emergencies for Pre-Hospital Providers).

Much like an infantry unit calls in artillery support, when outnumbered by the enemy, a medic can call an ER doc on the radio if he or she is stumped on a call. I'd rather pass the buck than make the wrong choice of treatment. The voice on the other end of the radio is making a hell of a lot more money than me, and sometimes I need to make them earn it.

Some patients are so critical that there's no time to call and you must act quickly. This is where the experience part of the job kicks in, and we go with our gut instinct. Unlike the hospital, on the street there's no doctor behind us, no safety net. We must believe in ourselves and have confidence in the decisions we make.

Needless to say, paramedics are grossly underpaid and overworked. What's worse is that we are told nothing can be done about it, and that is total smoke screen bullshit.

I think the people in position to increase salaries of paramedics, such as local politicians and director heads, often feel the change is more than justified. However, such change might affect *their* personal incomes, so they don't push it.

"Para-medicine is still a relatively new health care field compared to nursing, and so it doesn't warrant the same pay," is the common excuse we hear. How long can they milk this? Paramedics have been around for the last 40 years and continue to evolve. The actual job of a paramedic is broadening every year with more responsibilities being thrust upon us and no pay adjustment in sight. Pretty soon instead of folks going to the local free clinic, they'll just go to the closest ambulance down the street. This totally undermines what EMS is all about.

Every day the TV news deals with public health care reform and how everyone deserves to be able to have health care. Are they fucking blind? There already is free public health care, and the honest taxpaying citizen continues to pay for it!

Now, what I'm about to write is going to piss off some people, especially the liberal Hollywood types, but I don't give a damn. These people live in their cushioned, pampered, multimillionaire worlds while preaching to us lower class commoners how the rest of the world should be. To hell with them! If they care so much about us, why are movie and concert ticket prices so high? Most of the more outspoken ones don't even live in this country, but in places like France and Italy—and they still bitch. Screw them.

54 TONES

CHAPTER 8

Now back to the public health care situation. In my career I have never seen anyone refused treatment, at least in the form of emergency care, be it in an ER or EMS. Everyone is treated the same regardless of lifestyle or financial standing. There's a large population of illegal immigrants from South America in my town, and they receive the same care as the ultra rich, retired corporate CEO from New York. The only difference is that only one of these would actually be expected to pay the bill. Guess which one? Although I could easily use several personal examples, I'll just focus on the one that comes to mind the most. Self-appointed saviors of humanity might want to close their eyes at this point. That was another liberal slam, sorry.

There was a guy from Mexico that my co-workers and I used to run on daily. We would always find him drunk, staggering, and sometimes passed out at the same street corner. Other than being a drunken waste of human flesh, there was never anything medically wrong with him. He'd usually be seen wearing the ER admission bracelet from his last visit. There's nothing like a patient who has already been tagged by the hospital before he even gets there.

Not only was this guy in this country illegally, but he had no ID card and no health insurance. The cops didn't want to deal with him so they would always pawn him off on EMS. At times I feel like we are a human garbage disposal. This guy would always spit at us and curse us out in Spanish. I'd be lying if I said the thought of driving him to another town and dumping him off didn't cross my mind. Instead we would transport him to the local hospital like anyone else. He ran up hundreds of thousands of dollars in EMS and hospital bills. Did he ever send you a thank you card? I know I never got one, and you and I paid his bills. That's to say, the ones that weren't written off.

On one occasion while I was dealing with this poor soul, a cardiac arrest call came in just down the street and I couldn't respond. Several minutes after the call went out, another unit went blaring by en route to it, while I was still dealing with this drunk. On a code, seconds can mean the difference between life and death. Maybe it's just me, but something's not right with this picture. Eventually this guy was deported back to Mexico after being arrested for grabbing a nurse's ass in the ER.

What took so long, and why hadn't the *powers that be* put an end to this bullshit sooner? I guess it will take themselves or someone they care about having to wait for the next available ambulance before they open their eyes. It shouldn't have to come to that. Changes can be made, but nobody in a position to make them seems to care.

Saying nobody cares is an overstatement. There are a lot of us lower tier medical professionals who do, but again, nobody wants to hear from us. The rule is "Keep your mouth shut and run the calls."

As I review what I've written so far, I realize that I come off as extremely bitter, so let me make this perfectly clear. I still like the feeling of being able to help somebody who really needs it, and I have never let my personal feelings interfere with my treatment of a patient. I don't care about anyone's race, creed, religion or any of that. If a person is in need of medical care, I give him the best that I can. It is how we are paid, perceived, and treated that gets me down. EMS workers are long overdue the respect they deserve. I doubt it will come during my career, but hopefully it will change for the future generations of emergency workers.

58 TONES

CHAPTER 9

There are a lot of positive aspects of this job I need to mention. They include the friendships developed and the strong sense of brotherhood we share. There's a bit of an "us versus them" mentality among us.

Emergency workers are a strange and eclectic bunch. We've chosen a profession that places us in the most surreal situations. We see some of the darkest, disturbing, and most painful moments encountered in life as well as some of the most beautiful. We see lives enter this world as well as leave.

I can truly say that I love these EMS people, and I'm sure I will repeat this again before I'm done. Even though the odds are against them, they still get on the trucks and run the calls. In the past, I've had Public Safety Department heads say that monkeys could do our jobs or since we only went to a *trade school* and not to college that we should be paid less. One department head even called us *inmates in an asylum*. I could be wrong, but statements like those aren't very motivating. To this day I've never seen a monkey bring someone in cardiac arrest back to life—but what do I know, I only went to trade school. What makes this even worse is one of these guys is a retired millionaire with no experience in EMS and our county is paying him six figures a year.

I know everyone, regardless of their line of work, has to deal with an asshole boss at some point in time. That's just life. The fact that there seems to be such an abundance of hypocritical, arrogant, and condescending people holding high-level positions in my field amazes me. How are people who don't give a shit about the ones who work for them able to sleep at night?

Lord knows I'm not a saint. Hell, I've messed up a lot of things in my life. Before the Army I was an awful son who didn't care much about anything but me. In my teen years I caused my folks a lot of heartache. Making peace with my father before he died is one of my biggest accomplishments.

Before I started working with EMS, I began dating a medic whom I had ridden with as a student. I loved her. As I mentioned earlier, I've never been good at relationships. I've just never understood how or why a girl could care about me, considering the fact that in my man whore days I treated girls like a piece of ass.

She cared about me anyway, even after I told her that I had never been one to settle down. Being with her taught me that getting to know a woman for who she is was more important than how she looked or how she was in bed. My guy friends will think I'm full of shit but it's true, and just for the record, my girl was beautiful.

We used to take walks on the beach and hang out all the time. She even convinced me to go to church with her. One Christmas I went with her to visit old folks at a nursing home. She brought her dog along and she'd put fake reindeer antlers on its head. She had such a kind heart, and we could talk about anything, but she also had inner demons which I suppose we all do.

After a brief split, we had gotten back together. She was a bipolar depressive, and there were times when she just needed her space—but then we would get back together again. We did that three or four times, and the last time we got back together, I was really determined to make things work. At the time, she had just left EMS for a career in nursing and I thought everything was going great, but I was *so* wrong. One night while I was at work, she committed suicide.

I had missed all the signs. I will carry that guilt with me to the grave. After her death I was such a coward I couldn't even bring myself to attend the funeral. I miss her deeply and think about her every day. The loss of her was devastating to me.

62 TONES

CHAPTER 10

I've given you some background about myself, my job and the kind of environment I work in. You've heard of some of the messed up things that go on in the medical field and how nothing is being done to fix them, plus the general mentality of the public towards EMS. It's time for me to start my reflection of some of the most unique calls I've had over the years.

Some are funny, some sad, and some are just so absurd you probably won't believe them. I assure you, they are all true. Not all of these were run with the same partner, as over the years I've worked with several. Try to forget everything EMS-related you've seen in the movies, and just imagine you're in my shoes.

It was 5 a.m. on a Christmas morning some years ago, and I was sound asleep at one of our stations located at a firehouse. Boom! Boom! Boom! A loud knock on my bunk room door woke me up.

A firefighter told me a man had just come to the station, and he said there was a dead baby down the street. I got my partner up and we responded with firefighters to the address the man had given.

We followed a dirt road to a group of rundown mobile homes. Upon our arrival, a group of what I can only describe as inbred looking rednecks gathered outside one of the trailers. My partner on this call was new, and she had a small baby of her own, so I told her to wait outside while I went inside first. It's not that this type of situation is easy on me. It's just that I don't have any children and my partner did. I didn't want her to see anything she didn't have to.

Entering the home I found a young pregnant woman in her husband's arms, and at least four other small children running around. A small, crooked tree with Christmas lights stood in the corner of a disheveled front room. The husband directed me to a dimly lit back room. On the bed I found an 18-month-old baby boy facedown. As I touched him, I already knew it was too late. He was cold and stiff with rigor mortis.

The father told me there was no heat in the home, so the whole family slept together. He must have rolled on top of his son. I approached the mother, who was crying uncontrollably, and told her that I was very sorry but there was nothing I could do.

By this time law enforcement had arrived, which is routine. As I was explaining to the officer what had happened, the husband again hugged his wife and said,

"Don't worry babe, you still gotta handful of young'uns to cuddle with."

I briefly glanced up at the couple with what had to be a look of disbelief and again offered my condolences before leaving. On the way back to the station I told my partner what had happened without going into too much detail, and she thanked me for letting her stay outside.

"Merry Christmas," I replied.

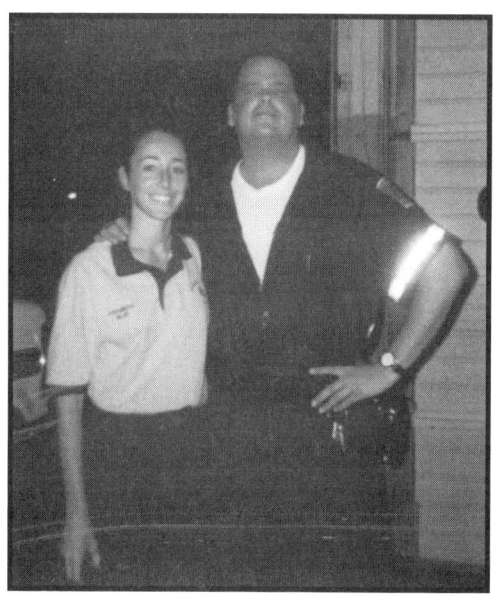

Jackie and me after returning from a call.

For some reason I've had a lot of unique calls during the holidays. On another Christmas day, my partner and I were called to a suspected DOA (Dead on Arrival). An elderly man with a thick southern drawl met us at the front door of his house. He told us he thought his sister was dead. Entering the house there was the familiar smell of mothballs, which for some reason seems to be in all elderly homes, overpowering the scent of coffee coming from the kitchen. An elderly woman was lying on the living room floor, and she appeared to have died during the night.

After informing the brother that his sister had passed away, we sat at the kitchen table and got information for our report while awaiting law enforcement. The man told us that his sister had come down from Tennessee for the holidays, and she had not been feeling well. While we were writing our report, he offered us coffee, which we respectfully declined.

"I'd better call my other sister and let her know that Agnes has passed away," he said while he dialed the phone … "Hello … Ruth? This is Frank … Merry Christmas, Agnes is dead."

My partner and I looked at each other, trying not to laugh. Those old southern folk just don't mince words; they get *right* to the point.

People react differently when confronted with an emergency. Some remain relatively calm, while others will become hysterical. I try not to judge, but when someone is totally losing it on a scene that turns out to be a non-emergency, it baffles me. I was with my old partner, Jackie, who I loved, even though she was like an annoying little sister. We responded to a call on

Christmas Eve morning where dispatch was advising that a hysterical husband was saying that his wife was in Cardiac Arrest and he was attempting CPR.

On calls like these, the fire department automatically responds with us for extra hands. This was another early morning call, and the man met us outside crying and begging us to save his wife. Following him inside, I asked where she was, and he pointed to a couch.

Now I know I only have a trade school education, but it didn't take long to deduce that there was nobody on the couch.

"Sir, there's no one on your couch. Where is your wife?" I asked.

The man looked at me and began laughing. "Oh no, I did it again," he said. "My wife left me years ago and sometimes I have dreams about her. I must have had another one."

The crazy part of this was that he had actually been doing chest compressions on the couch cushion. Oh well, another piece of furniture saved. I had another partner I worked with for about two years and we became good friends. One Christmas Day we were working in the zone where his grandfather lived. His family was having a big dinner and invited us over. As we were getting ready to go to his grandfather's, we got a call to back up another unit on an MVC.

This wreck was in the rural part of the county and it took us a while to get there. Arriving, we found a smoldering, overturned car wrapped around a tree, along with the first unit, which had arrived before us. It had a severely burned female in back. The medevac helicopter that had been called for the burn victim had actually beaten us there.

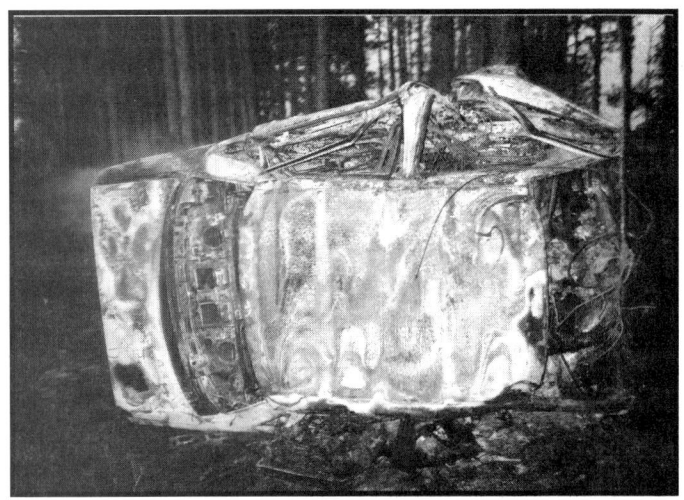

Christmas MVC in which father and daughter were killed.

As it turned out, there was just one patient, and I could hear her screaming about a baby as she was being transferred to the medevac crew. After the helicopter took off, my partner and I walked over to the car that had earlier been engulfed in flames.

The car, which was now extinguished, was still smoking and we could see the driver burned to a crisp and pinned under the car. We walked around the car looking for a baby, and fortunately, we didn't find one. I kicked something on the ground, and at first thought it was a piece of wood. Soon, I realized it was the driver's burned, amputated foot. We found out later that this had been a father and his adult daughter on their way to their own family Christmas.

After clearing the call, we went over to my buddy's grandfather's place for dinner, and what a spread they had set up. There was baked ham, mashed potatoes, and all the trimmings. My partner's mom was there, and with a curious look on her face, she asked if we had already eaten because we smelled like barbecue.

We didn't have the heart to tell her where the smell had come from, and we sat in a corner and quietly ate our dinner as the rest of his family gathered and listened to Christmas music. Even now the smell of baked ham makes me think of that day.

70 TONES

CHAPTER 11

Like a few of the calls I've just mentioned, some are confusing and you just have to deal with them. I was on an MVC a few years ago that had a confusing outcome.

I was working a swap day for one of my friends, which means I was working for him one day and he would pay me back by working one of my scheduled days. My unit was sent to a call on the interstate highway for an MVC. We were informed, en route, that there were multiple patients, including at least one child.

No matter what type of call you respond to, and I don't care who you are or how long you have been on the job, when it's a bad call and you're told that there is a child involved, your heart speeds up a little. Arriving on scene around midnight, it looked as if a bomb had exploded. Our headlights shined on a state trooper performing CPR on a small child, maybe three or four years old. There was debris everywhere, and at least four mangled vehicles spread across the highway. I told my partner to check out the other cars. I approached the small boy who was lying on the road as I radioed for additional units.

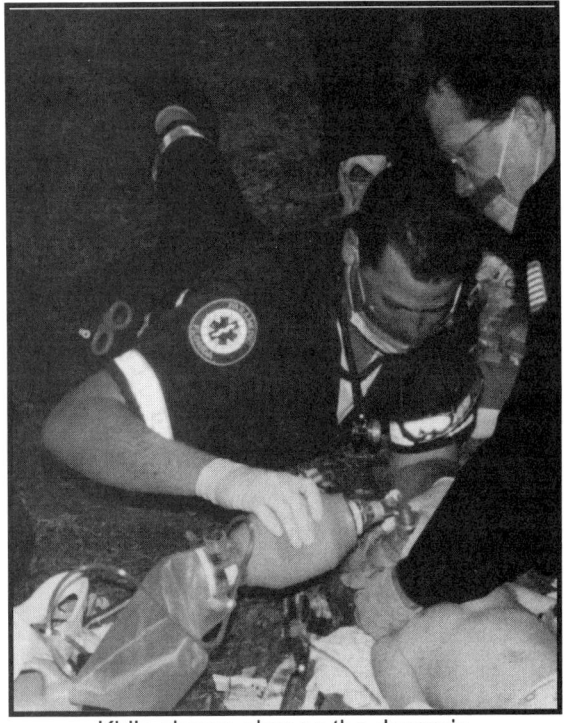

Kid's always change the dynamic.
Here I'm ventilating a little girl before intubation after she was hit by a car. Photo by Mark Skukowski. From authors collection.

The child was obviously dead from massive head trauma, but for some reason I told the trooper to keep doing CPR until I could get back to him. I then moved from car to car and assessed the other patients.

An elderly woman was trapped in one vehicle with both of her feet nearly amputated. In another car I found a man grossly trapped and barely breathing. It was from his car that the boy had been ejected.

As I was calling dispatch with a situation report, my shift captain arrived and I turned command of the scene over to him after summarizing the situation for him. I returned to the trooper who was still doing CPR on the boy and told him to stop because nothing more could be done. I'd run a lot of calls with this guy and he was as tough as nails, but seeing him choke up really got to me. I couldn't dwell on that though, I had a job to do and other patients to treat.

With my backup units arriving, I focused on the man who was trapped. The car he was in was crushed around him, and the fire crew had to cut it apart. While he was still pinned inside, I managed to climb in behind him through the broken rear windshield and start an IV. After several minutes, the fire crew, led by my friend Bobby, got him extricated and secured on a spinal immobilization board.

He was semiconscious and I had to RSI him. RSI or Rapid Sequence Intubation is where we administer medications to temporarily paralyze a patient to allow him to be intubated. After paralyzing the patient, we can place a breathing tube in their trachea and breathe for them.

In my town the closest trauma center is 50 miles away so any critical trauma patients are flown there.

Trauma centers are regular hospitals with specialized surgeons and staff on call for serious trauma.

As the helicopter took off with my patient, I went to one of my backup units to see if they needed any help. They had the woman whose feet were pretty much torn off. While they were dealing with her airway, they asked if I could start an IV for them, which I did. After everything was said and done, we had flown out three critical patients. Two of those died. In the end, three people were killed and several others injured. The man I treated was the grandfather of the boy that was killed, and he was high on drugs while driving the wrong way on the interstate. He was the second to die and the elderly woman passed away several days later.

This was a screwed up call for everyone involved. Not from an emotional point of view, but a logistical one. The first fire crew on scene had a mechanical failure with their extrication equipment, so a second crew had to do the cutting. It didn't really matter because the guy entrapped was so severely injured that he was going to die anyway. Because a child had been killed, my captain had us attend a CISD (Critical Incident Stress Debriefing) which is standard procedure. It was three in the morning, and that trooper and I were the only ones who had dealt with the child. I wasn't really thinking about it, and everyone else was tired, so the whole debriefing was a waste of time. These debriefings usually have someone who wasn't even on the scene telling you how you should feel. Sometimes these are people not even involved in the emergency world at all. I truly appreciate the fact that these folks want to help, but no thanks. They haven't walked the walk.

A few weeks after the call, my captain told me I was getting an award for my actions on that night. "I'm getting an award for *what*?" I asked. He told me our chief thought it would be good PR (public relations) to have the press see me and my co-workers get an award.

This is where the confusion I mentioned earlier comes in. Although I didn't want it or understand why I was receiving it, I was given an award for a call where every patient I'd touched had died. Is that fucked up, or what? That's like getting the Lombardi Trophy after your team *lost* the Super bowl. There have been calls where either one of my peers or I have gone above and beyond what is expected without getting the slightest nod—but if the higher-ups see a PR chance, everyone is a hero.

I'm sure everyone has either seen a movie or heard of a story about someone pulling a victim from a burning car. Believe it or not, I had one of those calls. Arriving on the scene of an MVC, we found a car that had hit a tree head-on and its engine compartment was on fire. I could see the driver slumped over the steering wheel, and as the unit slowed, I jumped out of the passenger side where I was sitting. In doing so, the door flew forward, cracking the side of the hood. I ran to the car and found an unresponsive male who weighed about 250 pounds. After unfastening the seat belt, I dragged him about 30 feet from the car before my partner and a paramedic student I was mentoring got to us.

I left them with the patient and ran back to the truck to retrieve the fire extinguishers. I managed to put out the fire just as the fire department arrived. At first I thought the patient was drunk, but he turned out to be diabetic.

Did I get a thank you card from the patient? No. Did I get an award from the chief? Nope. What I *did* get to do was write an incident report for cracking the hood of the truck. I guess the rest wasn't *PR worthy*.

Another call that wasn't PR worthy was the time my partner and I stopped to help a little girl who was hit by a pickup truck during a brawl outside a pool hall. Our unit was out of service after running a very bloody call, and we were returning to the station to clean up. It was about 2 a.m. and my partner on this call was Gene, who also happened to be one of my best friends.

Gene was a big guy who had a part time job bouncing at one of the local strip clubs. I'm six foot two and weigh 220 pounds, but he made me look tiny. While he made a lot more money bouncing than working in

EMS, bodybuilding and thumping heads were only hobbies to him. He was also a damned good EMT.

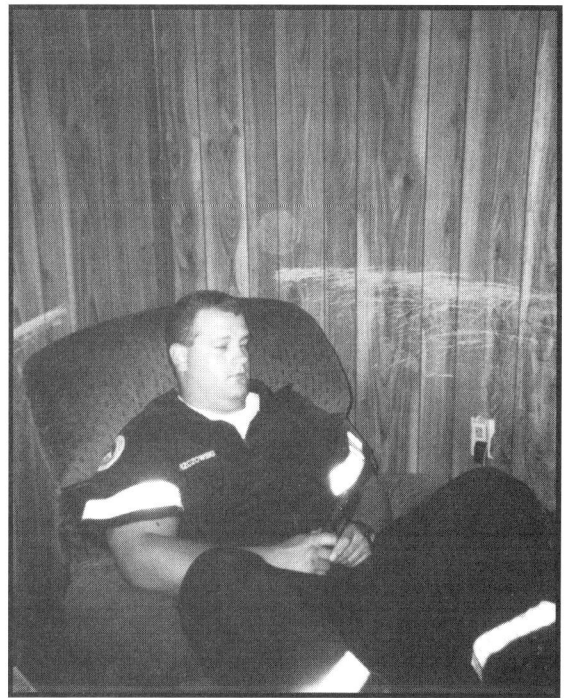
Gene snoozing after running calls all night.

As we were driving back to station, he noticed a large group of people fighting outside a pool hall. We told dispatch what was going on and turned around to watch the fight. I could lie and say we were going to see if anyone was hurt, but the truth is we wanted to watch a bunch of drunks beat the shit out each other. Pulling into the parking lot, people started flagging us down and a young Hispanic woman walked toward us with a limp little girl in her arms.

It turns out a group of rednecks got into it with a group of Mexicans and the child was hit by a vehicle trying to leave. Realizing that this was more than just a bar fight, I told dispatch to step up law enforcement and respond another ambulance. Dispatch advised me that they were now receiving multiple calls on the fight including shots fired—and they advised us to leave the scene.

Ignoring dispatch, we got out and went over to the woman with the child. The little girl was unresponsive with a large gash to her head. As soon as I took her from the mother, the mother collapsed, cracking her head on the pavement. As I held the child, the mother started seizing on the ground.

Gene was moving toward the woman when gunshots erupted from the crowd in the parking lot. Placing the child on the ground, I tried to cover her up as best I could with my body while Gene stood between us and the crowd.

"Back the fuck up!" he shouted without even flinching. I was protecting the kid, and he was protecting *us* as he told dispatch, "More shots fired!"

Within seconds, the first cop arrived, and it looked like something from a movie as the patrol car slid to a stop. At this point the crowd was easily a hundred, and the lone female cop got out with her weapon drawn. "Everybody, back the hell up!" she ordered. I must admit, despite the situation, as I watched her, I was aroused.

Soon more cops arrived as well as my second unit, and fortunately nobody had been shot. There ended up being several patients. Two were flown to a trauma center and they all survived.

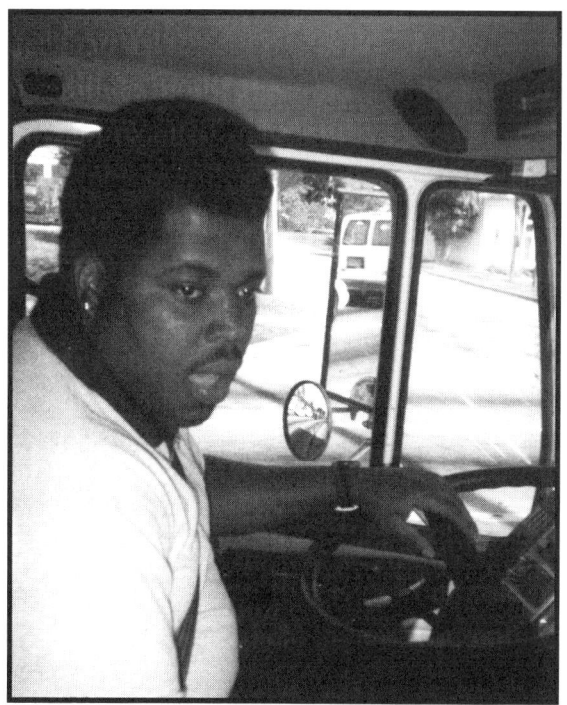

Dequan, co-founder of the famous BBQ's.

After the call I was verbally reprimanded for endangering my crew by not leaving the scene when dispatch advised that shots had been fired. In part, I guess I was guilty, but leaving that little girl was not an option for Gene and me. Even to this day, we both agree that if the same scenario happened again, we would still react the same way.

As was the case with the last call I described with Gene, I've had the opportunity over the years to run calls with some of my closest friends. Every football season I have BBQ's at my house where I have my best friends over, most being from EMS. It's like our own little family within a larger one. We watch the game, drink, eat, and vent any frustrations we might have with the knowledge that *what's said at Dave's, stays at Dave's*.

We are able to talk and listen to each other when nobody else will. We try to keep work talk to a minimum so as to not totally bore our non-EMS friends. My buddy Dequan (or DQ as we call him) and I started these parties years ago, after working together for the first time. When you're stuck with someone for 24 hours, you find yourselves talking about all kinds of stuff, and we talked about football and BBQ. Thus, the birth of our parties took place, and over the years we have perfected them.

DQ and I were working together one time when we were given a call to back up another unit that was working an MVC. A car had hit a young deaf man on a bicycle, and we found the initial crew trying to intubate the patient in the middle of the road. It was night time, and a light rain was starting to fall as we walked up to the scene. This guy was a mess. He was unconscious with massive head trauma including a shattered jaw and sliced throat just below the jaw and above the Adam's apple.

The first medic on scene was unable to intubate and asked me if I wanted to try. I subsequently lay down on the wet road behind the patient's head to attempt the intubation. I still remember the smell of rain mixing with the strong metallic smell of the blood—and I hate the smell of blood.

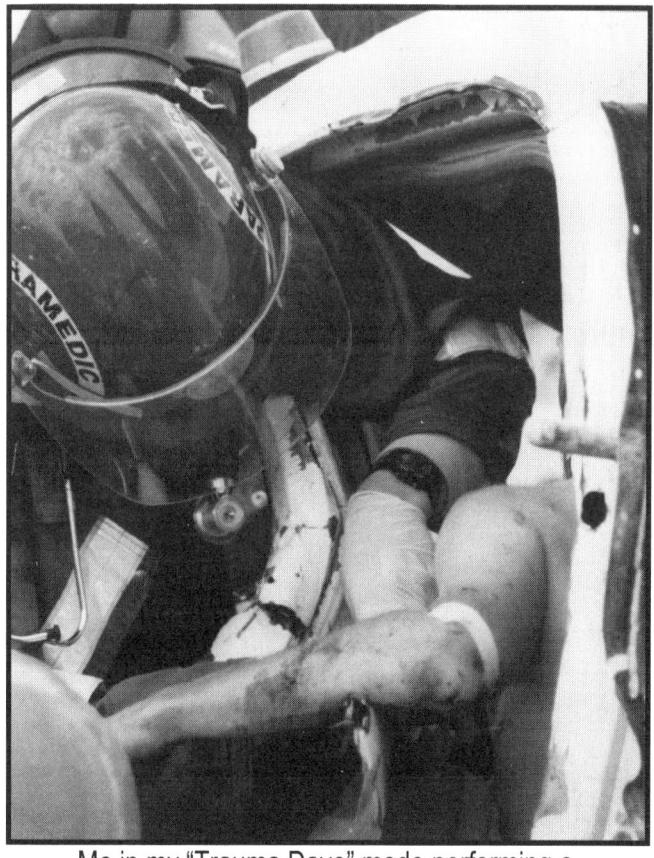

Me in my "Trauma Dave" mode performing a chest decompression on entrapped MVC patient.
Photo by Mark Skukowski. From authors collection.

A piece of broken jaw bone had lacerated the underside of his tongue, and it was hanging out of his mouth like a large dog's tongue. I slid the laryngoscope into his mouth and attempted to visualize the vocal cords so I could push the airway tube through them and we could breathe for him. I couldn't see shit because of all the blood and that fucking tongue.

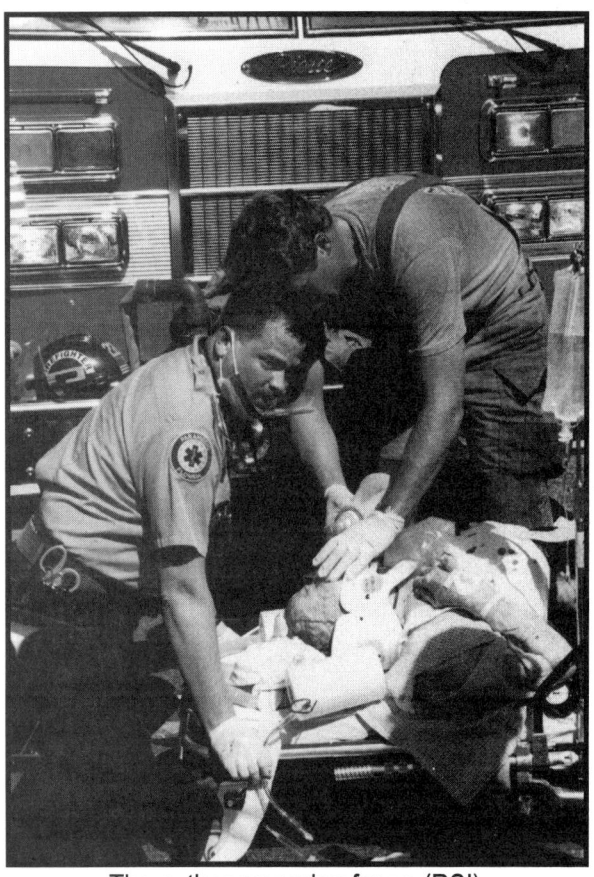

The author preparing for an (RSI) Rapid Sequence Intubation.
Photo by Mark Skukowski. From authors collection.

While I was still looking, DQ tapped me on the shoulder, and calmly said, "Hey Bro. Check it out," as he pointed to the patient's throat. I looked up and noticed the laryngoscope blade, which is a six-inch-long crescent-shaped piece of steel with a light on the end, coming out of the slit in the patient's throat. It kind of reminded me of a fish on a hook.

"What the fuck?" I said in disbelief, and just then the patient coded. Hearing the patient had gone into cardiac arrest, the medevac helicopter that had been responding cancelled. The odds of resuscitating a trauma code are extremely small.

We loaded the patient in the truck and sped off for one of the local ER's. While en route, and with no other options, I performed a cricothyrotomy. This is an invasive procedure where an incision is made through the cricothyroid membrane. This membrane is just below the Adam's apple, and once the incision is made, if done correctly, an airway tube can be placed into it allowing us to get air into the lungs. It is rare that this procedure is needed, but in my career I have performed four of them. After the airway was secured, we got pulses back on the patient as we pulled into the ER parking lot. The staff was expecting a trauma code, but they got a rude awakening when we rolled in the door, and I informed them we had a return of pulses.

This staff was not accustomed to getting major trauma because we fly out the most critical patients. They started freaking out. Moments earlier two medics were treating this guy alone in the back of a cramped ambulance without freaking out, and now, practically the entire ER staff was tripping over themselves.

I guess keeping your head while those around you are losing theirs, only counts for medics. The doctor who was in charge was the only one who had her shit together. By this time one of my supervisors had arrived and was standing next to me as the ER staff went to work.

"Who did the crich?" the doctor asked as she wiped her brow.

"I did," I replied while nudging my supervisor with my elbow.

"Good job. I couldn't have done better myself!" she exclaimed.

I felt pretty good about that, if only for myself, because naturally I didn't even get a pat on the back from my administration. In the end, the young man died—big surprise. But, because we helped keep him alive, they were able to harvest his organs. Some sick and dying people benefited from this young man's misfortune and the fact that we did not give up. Hopefully, reading about this call will provide a lesson to others—be an organ donor.

After returning to station, we were given another MVC call just a few blocks away from the last one, and it involved the same guy who had hit the bicycle. Talk about dumb luck, this poor bastard had only made it a couple of blocks before he got into another wreck. Just like the first one, it wasn't his fault and he wasn't injured.

"Fuck it!" he said. "I'm walking home."

Who could blame him?

Speaking of blocks or streets, I have three in my regular zone I run calls on all the time. I've named these streets Dumb, Dumber, and Dumbest. Every call I run on these streets involves some level of brainless moron. I will never understand how the majority of idiots in a town can all end up in the same neighborhood. That's not saying there aren't more of them spread throughout town, there's just a larger accumulation of them in this area.

Regardless of what dispatch tells me, if I'm running a call on one of those streets, I know it will be really stupid. Just a couple weeks ago I ran a call on Dumbest Street involving a 20-something white trash female. Her boyfriend, Bobby Lee or Billy Jo or *whatever-his-name*, had beaten the shit out of her. Her front teeth were knocked out and she was spitting blood as she pleaded with the cop on scene not to arrest her man.

"He loves me! Please don't arrest him! He didn't mean it!"

Oh yeah, just look at the love all over her face, not to mention she's pregnant and trying to smoke a cigarette with her bloody, toothless gums. That baby doesn't have a chance, and in twenty years someone will be running calls on its dumb ass. People like this remind me of great white sharks' teeth. If one falls out, there are rows behind it ready to fill its space.

CHAPTER 12

Ignorance, stupidity, the nature of aging, and just plain bad luck equals job security in the EMS world. Sometimes things happen that just can't be avoided, but then there are the *frequent flyers*, and they represent one of the worst parts of the job. These types include hypochondriacs, drug seekers, homeless, and some who just thrive on attention.

Before I go further into this subject, I must point out that over the years I have met some truly awesome homeless people, who have just been screwed over by life. There was one homeless man in particular that I ran on several times who was a very kind and gentle person. He never once called for himself, but people would see him sleeping and instead of asking him if he was all right, they would call 911. He always apologized for wasting our time, and I would tell him not to worry.

I don't live far from the area where he would hang out. Whenever I would see him either on or off duty, I would buy him something to eat and a bottle of water. I wouldn't give him money because I was afraid the other homeless might rob him or he would waste it on booze.

I found out from a friend at work that he had passed away, and that really bummed me out. I wish I would have gotten off my high horse, sat down, and talked to him. I'm sure he would have had a story to tell.

Life is a bunch of wishes, and I sometimes wish everyone could see it through a medic's eyes. By writing this book, even some of my closest friends are seeing a side of me they didn't know existed. I've earned a reputation of being a hard ass, but like everyone, I am only human. That's not saying I won't hesitate to speak my mind when dealing with an asshole, especially frequent flying assholes—and yes, that has gotten me in trouble. I try to keep my mouth shut but sometimes it's tough. It may be hard to believe, but I'm not a very politically correct individual. Ha!

Drug seekers are the worst, and we have several where I work. There's one in particular I have run on no less than 50 times, and I can honestly say that this crazy bitch is the most annoying person I have ever dealt with. Every hospital in five counties knows her for drug-seeking and turns her away, but she keeps calling.

Let me digress. *Drug seekers* are individuals who are addicted to some form of medication, mostly pain killers, and go from hospital to hospital looking for a fix. They can't afford the drugs on the street so they call *America's Yellow Cab*, aka ambulance, and go to an ER faking some sort of pain.

Back pain is the most popular, and it usually takes three to four visits before the hospital catches on. Once that happens, they request another hospital until they abuse them all. You've got to love our health care system.

Back to my favorite customer—who all of the veteran crews in my service have run on at least once. She seemed to follow me like the plague and always ended up in the same part of town that I was working. Fake slip and falls, abdominal pain, back pain, and even a so-called spider bite to the ass—with her I heard it all.

Everyone has complained about her, even the hospitals, and nothing has been done for whatever reason. I mean *really*, why should anyone in a position to make change get their hands dirty? I told her the last time I ran on her that she would never get into one of my trucks again unless she was in a body bag, and I even suggested which bridge she should jump off. I still see her in the ER from time to time, and as far as I know, she walked there.

This is a nationwide burden on the health care system, and in my eyes it is a crime. These abusers should be punished for what they do, but instead of fines or jail time, they're given a pass. I don't think I'll ever understand the reasoning for that.

It's like the career criminals. They continue committing crimes no matter how many prison terms they serve. Seriously, how many times should innocent people suffer because of liberal laws? These thugs obviously don't care about you and me and should be given life at hard labor, or even better—they should be *shot*. Enough is enough.

I know some people believe in rehabilitation, and they think these criminals had tough childhoods which has caused them to inflict pain and suffering on others. I wish these people would take off their rose-colored glasses and view reality. Have you ever seen the body of someone who was brutally murdered? I have and I can tell you that the ones who did the killing could give a shit about rehabilitation. They don't care about hurting innocents. Judges and politicians have screwed this wonderful country up over the years, and they need to try to fix it or get the hell out of office. That's my opinion anyway.

CHAPTER 13

In my last rant about frequent flyers I mentioned body bags. My EMS service doesn't actually pick up dead bodies, but some of us used to do it as a part time job. I did it for about a year, and it was easy money. There would be two of us on call with pagers for 24 hours, and most of the time we didn't get any calls. If no calls came in, we still got three hours of overtime pay—not bad.

Unfortunately, there *were* times we did get a page, and sometimes the job was downright nasty. When you arrive at a scene to find two week's worth of newspapers outside, you know it's going to be a Stinker (decomposing body). Trust me. That's a smell you should try to avoid. I would describe it as the smell of rotting road kill multiplied by a thousand.

Not all of the body removal calls were bad, that is, smell wise. I had one where my partner for the day and I had to pick up some guy in his forties who committed suicide by drug overdose. A cop led us upstairs to the body. We put a sheet over the guy and zipped him up in the body bag. These bags are dark green and made of a durable plastic with carrying handles. Now, this body weighed about 200 pounds, and my partner for the day was a little scrawny guy. I had the bottom half while we were moving backwards, carrying it down the stairs. As we did this, I could hear voices in the room at the bottom of the stairs.

Trying not to drop him, I suddenly noticed a thumping sound, and I realized my weak-assed partner was letting the head bang on the steps. Coming around the corner at the end of the stairway, I found family members had gathered in the living room, and they started freaking out. I felt like I was part of the *Three Stooges* minus Moe.

I've seen a lot of graphic trauma scenes over the years, but my last body removal call took the cake. It's one thing to see a mangled body on an EMS scene because you just pronounce them dead and walk away, but on body removal, you have to pick it up along with any separated parts.

It was a Sunday morning in late January and I was feeling great. My New Year's resolution had been to quit smoking and drinking. It was so far, so good. At about 10 a.m. the pager went off. I called dispatch for the address, and picked up the body removal van. My partner was supposed to meet me at the scene but he never showed up, so one of my EMS supervisors was on his way to help me.

While I was waiting I asked the cops on scene what was going on, and they started laughing at me. I knew these pricks, and they were getting a kick out of something.

"You got one of those fancy plastic suits and rubber boots?" they asked. "You're going to need them."

Thinking these guys were just messing with me, I headed towards the house. Inside I found an older cop who was a CSI type. This guy wasn't laughing, and he informed me that the victim shot himself in the head with a deer rifle. He pointed to a closed door at the end of a hallway.

As I got to the door, the hair on the back of my neck stood up. Still unsure if the guy's outside were fucking with me, I slowly opened the door, and the first thing I noticed was a nose with a partial upper lip and mustache on the floor. Looking up, I felt like I had walked into a scene from the *Texas Chainsaw Massacre*. This guy's head had exploded from the gas expansion coming from the barrel. He had sat at the edge of a bed and put the barrel of a 300 Winchester in his mouth. This was his friend's house and I guess he didn't want to make a mess so he had placed a towel on the floor. Naturally, the towel was the only thing in the room left unscathed.

After pulling the trigger with his big toe and his head blowing apart, the bullet went through the ceiling and exited the roof. The back of his head was stuck to a wall, and his brain was split in half, resting on his lap. From the top of the chin on up, there was nothing, and I noticed part of his lower jaw stuck to a ceiling fan that was slowly spinning. I could even see fillings in the teeth. The clothes hanging in the closet were splattered with blood and pieces of bone, and there was an ear lying on a flip flop.

My help finally arrived, and we slopped this lump of goo into a body bag and contemplated how we would gather the rest of the mess.

"I am not picking up this guy's fucking brain," I declared. The supervisor also refused. To the veteran crime scene cop with us, we must have looked like two school kids double-daring each other.

"Just give me some gloves! I'll do it!" he said, with a disgusted look on his face.

I held open a red bio-hazard trash bag as this guy went to work. There was a squishing sound as he picked up the brain parts and dropped them into the bag. I forgot to mention that there was that strong nauseating blood smell that I love so much permeating the room. While trying not to blow chunks, I watched the cop peel the skull cap off the wall and pick up the bigger parts from around the room. Once done, we put the bio-bag in with the rest of the body.

After delivering the body to the medical examiner's office and dropping off the van, I quit body removal. I stopped on the way home for a six pack of beer and some smokes. I'd had it!—So much for my New Year's resolutions. Nightmares come with the job, but earning extra money seeing things I didn't have to was for the birds.

Nightmares—I have had a few in my time, and at one point I contemplated seeing a shrink to have them analyzed. But what would they know? Unless they had been an EMS worker at some point in their lives, they wouldn't understand. I don't care how much education a person has or how many books by Freud they may have read. If they haven't walked the walk, they wouldn't understand.

I have found my solace talking to co-workers, and that has been the best therapy for me. I used to have a recurring dream, I'm not even sure if you could call it a nightmare. In my dream I would walk up to a bar and sit down. The bar was similar to the ones I hung out at during one of my tours in Korea when I was a soldier. After getting my beer, the person next to me would strike up a conversation, and we would talk about nonsensical bullshit. At some point during the dream, my bar mate would always ask, "Why me?" After that, I would turn and see a baby sitting next to me on a bar stool.

I could never figure out if the baby in the dream was a baby I saw die or one I helped deliver. Maybe it was one that wasn't born yet.

TONES

CHAPTER 14

I have played a part in several child births since I started with EMS. When I say *played a part*, I mean I have been there to help while the mom does all the work. Some EMS people will proclaim, "I delivered a baby last shift," or whenever. Bullshit! We simply play catch during the most natural occurrence of human existence.

Not all births are text book, and an example of this would be a breach birth where the legs deliver first. On this type of delivery the medic may have to help manipulate the baby out, but that is not advised. Unless obvious death is going to occur to the baby, we are trained to let nature take its course.

I still have a thank you card from a mother whose baby I helped deliver in the parking lot of the station I was working at. This happened about ten years ago, and I was at one of our stations located at a firehouse. I had just taken a bite from my sandwich when one of the fire guys walked in. He informed me that a car had pulled up in front of the station with a pregnant woman. Reluctantly putting my lunch down, I walked outside and found a very pregnant woman in a minivan.

With the firefighters help, we got her on the stretcher and into my truck. The stretcher was soaking wet because her water had broken already, and her contractions were 30 seconds apart. She was ready to pop. This was her fourth child, and she said it was coming soon. When it comes to a woman who's had several children with another one on the way, you forget the formalities and listen to her. Screw the paramedic patch on your shoulder—she's in charge.

While my partner attached the heart monitor to her and gave her oxygen via nasal cannula (plastic tubing that wraps around the ears and goes in the nose), I started an IV. She was moaning with each contraction, and they were getting closer as I looked between her legs.

This might be the point for a crude joke to some, but believe me, it's not. At this point I saw what appeared to be the crowning of the top of a head covered in hair. I turned away briefly to secure my IV, and when I turned back, I could no longer see the head.

Holy shit! Had the little guy squirted out while my back was turned? No, he had just retracted back inside. For a millisecond I thought he had shot out before I could catch him. Just then, one of the firefighters opened the back door and asked if he could help, and I said, "Keep your eyes on that," as I pointed between her legs. "If you see anything with more hair than that, let me know."

The baby was delivered shortly afterwards, and he and mother were fine. I would love to say that if it wasn't for my intense medical training, the baby might not have made it, but that wouldn't be the truth. Mom did all the work, and I just cleaned him up and cut the cord. Like childbirth, some things happen naturally and no fanfare is needed. A being is born, lives for however long, and then dies. That's just life. Why some people try to make it more than it is—confuses me.

I hate the phrase *Life is short*. If you die at five or die at 50, life is that long, so enjoy it. In the end we all die, and when it happens to us, if there is no afterlife, we won't know it anyway. Like I said before, I personally believe in an afterlife and considering what I've dealt with during this life so far, I'm sure the next will be great. I've earned it.

100 TONES

CHAPTER 15

As I'm writing this, it's that time of year when the snow birds start trickling down and that means twice as much work. For the most part they're all right, they are just old and nature is taking its course. Some, on the other hand, are total assholes and bring an arrogant *Northern attitude* with them.

"If we were in New York, you would have been here ten minutes ago" or "In Boston you people wouldn't make so much noise." Just once I wish I had the balls to tell them to stay up North. I know these old bastards are a boost for the local tourism industry, but it doesn't affect my paycheck at all. I haven't had a pay raise in going on five years, and the winter population keeps growing. If these people only knew that the more they bitch the less I care about them, maybe they would shut up. I will always treat them appropriately, but as far as going the extra mile—forget it.

There's a guy who works in my service from New York. He hates Boston, so that last dig is for him. Not only is he a co-worker, but he's also my neighbor.

One day my regular partner went home sick so I asked him to come in and work with me because I didn't want to get stuck with a rookie. He did, and jokingly he said that with us together on a truck, we were bound to get some kind of weird call. Naturally we did, and a couple of hours after he came into work, we got a call for a pedestrian accident just down the road from the station.

A young guy committed suicide by jumping in front of a car. Turns out this was the second time in a week he had tried this. Unfortunately, this time he did it right. Arriving on scene we found our patient face down on the road, and he had been hit and thrown so hard that his pants were twisted down around his ankles. Because we had gotten on scene so quickly, we found that he still had a pulse, which blew both of our minds because he was so fucked up. While we were packaging him for transport, he coded, so we took him to a local ER.

The ER doc pronounced him dead shortly after our arrival. An X-ray showed the only thing holding his head on was the skin. He had a closed decapitation. I'm not sure, but I think that has to be a first.

Back to old people bitching—and it's not just the Northern folks either. It seems to me that a lot of the elderly population, and it doesn't matter where they come from, are under the impression that those of us who are younger owe them something. It's not enough that we are trying to help them, but we are supposed to thank them at the same time.

I was brought up to respect my elders, and for the most part, I do. I can't tell you how many times I have thanked elderly veterans for their service to the country. At one point in time, they put their country before themselves, and as a veteran, I have a deep respect for them. When some of the older population, or any other patient for that matter, gives me attitude, I try to ignore it, and believe me, it's hard sometimes. The service I work for believes that the customer is always right, and they even refer to our patients as *customers*. I am not a cashier or sales rep. I don't have customers, I have patients—and *no,* they are *not* always right.

I had one old guy blow my partner and me shit one day because we had our emergency lights on when we pulled in front of his mobile home. He had called 911 because his wife had diarrhea, and he seemed more concerned with our entrance than his wife.

"I told the lady on the phone that I didn't want any lights or sirens. Now all my neighbors are watching!" he said in an angry tone. "That's what's wrong with this generation! You people don't listen and have no respect for what your elders have given you!"

I had had enough. "You're right, sir, we *do* owe you thanks. So, thanks to you and yours for our national debt, and the fact that because of your generation's mismanagement, there won't be any Social Security when I retire."

Man, was he pissed, I thought for sure he would call and complain, but I never heard anything about it. Maybe I had opened his eyes.

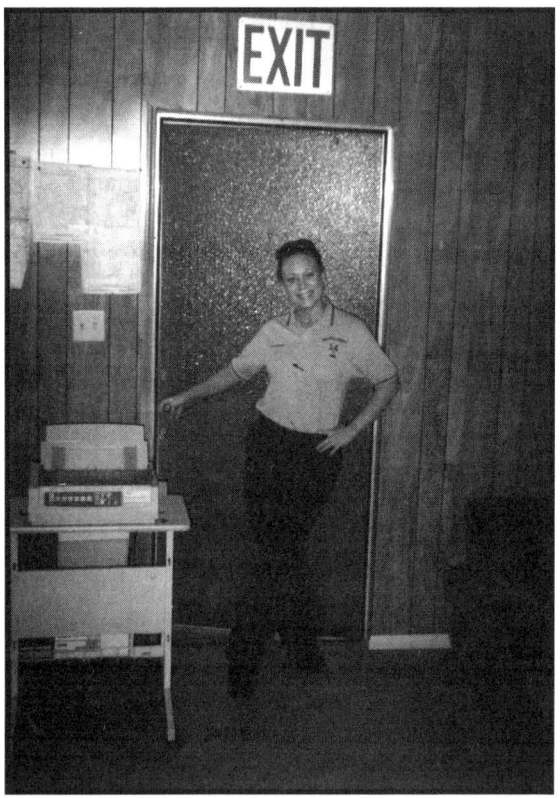

Michelle posing in our fancy doublewide station.

There are a lot of things to learn from the older part of our society, and I am a strong believer in studying history or it will repeat itself. Sometimes, even *they* do stupid things which go against all definitions of common sense.

One of my favorite partners was a girl named Michelle, and she and I ran a truly stupid geriatric call. This old man with emphysema, who obviously wasn't supposed to be smoking, decided to sit in his carport and light up. This guy wore a nasal cannula and was on oxygen 24/7. Now, I'm not trying to insult anyone's intelligence, but oxygen is extremely flammable.

Do you see where I'm going with this? You got it. As soon as he struck the match, the oxygen exploded. By the time we arrived, all of this man's hair was gone and the plastic cannula was melted to his face.

Even though he had second and third degree burns, as we approached him, he was trying to light another cigarette. This guy was in his eighties and didn't seem to give a shit about what had happened or show any signs of pain. It looked very painful to me, though, with the burnt skin hanging off and that melted cannula becoming part of his face.

"Just let me die," he said quietly.

I guess I couldn't blame him. He'd lived a long life and wanted it to end. Although I do believe in euthanasia, that's neither my call nor my job. We put him on a helicopter and flew him to a burn center where he eventually died. Not a very good death in my eyes, but he got his wish all the same.

106 TONES

CHAPTER 16

Learning from our seniors is one thing, but being shown a different perspective of life by a ten-year-old girl is something I never expected. We were called to a local pediatrician's office to transport a beautiful little girl to a children's hospital 50 miles away. She had a congenital pulmonary (lung) defect and needed specialized treatment.

During the transport I sat on the bench seat which is parallel to the stretcher. During a normal transport I sit in what is called the captain's chair located behind the patient's head, but, on this occasion, I wanted the girl to know she wasn't alone. I had her on oxygen and she didn't even flinch when I started an IV. I've had hardcore gang members cry like babies when I started an IV on them, but she didn't whimper. She was a real trooper and wise beyond her years.

I guess it's because I don't have children myself that I've always found it difficult to relate to them, but this little girl was different. She actually put me at ease. I don't know if it was because of all that she had been through with her affliction or maybe she was just smarter than the rest of us.

Instead of talking about *Sesame Street* or some other kid stuff, we talked about football—and that's something I can talk about with anyone. It turned out her favorite team was the same as mine, and she knew more about the team's stats than I did. Nearing the children's hospital, she asked how old I was and I told her, not knowing where she was going with the question.

She told me that she'd once overheard a doctor tell her mom that she most likely wouldn't live to see 20. "Sometimes I don't think life is fair. I'm just a kid," she said. "My friends are always having fun and I keep seeing doctors." That floored me. I mean, how could I respond to that?

I asked her if she wanted to hear some music and what her favorite station was. My partner, who was driving, turned the radio to her station and cranked it up as I moved to the captain's chair. Hoping the music would muffle any sounds I might make if I started crying, I didn't cry, but I damn sure teared up and realized how much I had been taking life for granted. This little girl had been through so much pain and was missing out on her childhood, yet she was so strong.

Through her, I realized that sweating the bullshit in life will get you nowhere. I still bitch about things—by now you already know that—but I will never take life for granted again. I don't know whatever happened to that little girl, but I hope she lives to be a Q-tip.

That's twice while writing this I've mentioned being bummed out or tearing up. I must come off as such a puss, and I'm sorry about that. Let me see if I can redeem myself with some of my less emotional moments.

My partner and I were eating dinner at this BBQ joint that had awesome baby back ribs. I was on my second or third rib when we got a call for a man threatening suicide with a gun. With that tangy sauce still on my lips, I grabbed my food and we responded to the call. Having polished off the ribs en route, I cleaned my hands with a baby wipe as we followed law enforcement into the subdivision where the call was located. Getting out of the unit, we heard the unmistakable sound of a gunshot, and a man came running out of the house.

"He just shot himself!" the man exclaimed as he slowed to a walk. He told us he was a neighbor and the man inside had terminal cancer. We followed the cop inside and found an elderly man in bed with smoke coming out of his mouth. For some reason, this made me think of the smoked ribs I had just eaten. The headboard was splattered with blood and brain matter, and the pistol he had used was still in his hand, resting on his chest.

The cop, who was turning green at this point, did a quick *about face* and walked outside. Knowing that any *death twitch* this guy might have could cause the weapon to discharge again, I removed it from his hand and checked for a pulse. I know that sounds stupid, with the brains being blown out and all, but it is procedure.

Fortunately he had no pulse so I pronounced him dead. By this time more cops had arrived, including one of their supervisors. After completing my report and giving my information over to law enforcement, we left the scene.

Not five minutes later, my own supervisor called me and said the police supervisor complained about me for having removed the gun from the man's hand. I explained how the call went down, and I explained that if the first cop had done his fucking job, I wouldn't have moved the weapon. Their job is to secure a scene for safety and if they won't do it, I will. I was more than willing to return to the scene to talk to the cops directly, but I was told to let it go. Oh well, I didn't give a shit in the first place.

I have actually had two suicides by shooting while I was trying to eat. The second one was a man who sat in a lawn chair outside his house and shot himself not once, but twice in the chest. I was at a popular fast food chicken place and had just gotten my chicken nuggets when the call came in. At this point I wouldn't blame you for calling this bullshit. I mean *really*, how many calls can a guy get while he's trying to eat?

I assure you they happened exactly how I described them. Murphy's Law, remember? We arrived at the same time as the fire department and police. Walking up to the man, I was just about to pronounce him dead when one of the firefighters said they felt a pulse. Shit! Now my nuggets were going to get cold. We placed him on the ground as I notified dispatch I had a Trauma Alert. The term Trauma Alert is used for critical trauma patients, and it lets dispatch know to respond a Medivac helicopter. This guy had two large caliber gunshot wounds to the center of his chest, and I couldn't believe he still had a pulse.

As we started to treat him, we lost pulses. *Thank God!* I thought to myself, and I cancelled the medevac.

When we have initiated treatment on a patient who codes and we don't believe they are viable, we have to call Medical Control for permission to stop working on them. Medical Control is any doctor at any of our local emergency rooms, and we give them a size-up of what's going on via radio telemetry.

Not wanting to let my nuggets get any colder, I walked back to the unit to make the call. Have you ever eaten cold nuggets? They suck. Using the radio in the front of the truck, I notified the closest ER that this patient had mortal wounds not consistent with life, and I wanted permission to cease any further efforts.

Waiting for their reply, I started eating my lunch and noticed the entire neighborhood was looking at me. That was awkward, but I didn't care, and I was given permission to pronounce the patient dead. Unlike TV where the medics would be crying in this situation, I didn't see it that way. The way I saw it—two things had been accomplished—a successful suicide and a lunch eaten.

I've talked about a lot of trauma calls, so let me mention a bizarre medical call I had. A man who was about my age, which would have been early thirties at the time, called 911 because he had a sudden onset of nausea and vomiting. In the service I'm in, each unit has a *charge paramedic* and an EMT. The EMT can also be a lesser-grade paramedic working in an EMT position.

What this really means is at least one of the crew must have passed a series of tests, including scenarios, with the medical director to be promoted to charge paramedic. Like the title says, he or she is in charge of the truck. On this particular call I was the senior charge medic, and my partner had just been promoted to charge.

The patient said he had been working in his yard all morning. Now, this was summer time in Florida, so the temperature was easily in the nineties, and I was thinking he was a possible heat casualty.

We asked the patient what exactly he had been doing, and he told us he had mowed his yard and was taking care of a weed problem. My partner, who was eager to start taking responsibility for calls, asked if he could have this one. I naturally said *yes,* because I can be lazy. We then started an IV on the patient and also administered supplemental oxygen and put him on the heart monitor.

Everything appeared normal as I drove us to the hospital, and all of a sudden all hell broke loose. My partner, in a panicked voice, asked me to pull over, something was wrong. As I got in the back of the unit, I noticed the monitor had gone from a normal rhythm into a very irregular one with multiple PVC's.

PVC's (Premature Ventricular Contractions) are when the heart's ventricles fire before they are supposed to in the normal sequence of the heart's beat. Having occasional PVC's is not uncommon. I have had them after drinking too much coffee in the morning.

This guy, on the other hand, was having about three or four every six seconds—not good. Multiple PVC's can lead to ventricular tachycardia (V-Tach) or ventricular fibrillation (V-Fib). Both of these can be fatal with V-fib presenting with cardiac arrest.

I asked the patient again exactly what he had been doing in the yard, and he began telling us he had also treated it for insects. He had mixed insecticide with his hands, and with that comment, I knew I was dealing with organophosphate poisoning. The phosphates are in the insecticides and they had been absorbed through his skin. Atropine is the name of the medication used to treat calls like this in a *normal* situation, but our patient was beyond that at this point. I told my partner to haul ass to the closest hospital and advised dispatch to have a firefighter meet us at an intersection coming up across the street from a fire station. I would need extra hands on this ride.

Just as I got the atropine ready, the patient's eyes rolled back and he went into V-fib. I immediately shocked his heart.

"Fuck!" he screamed, and he was suddenly back.

Stopping briefly, the firefighter jumped in, and I explained we might end up with a code. I have known this firefighter for years, and he was good at his job with the exception of being a brownnoser.

Racing to the hospital, I had to shock this gentleman several more times as well as administer medications trying to get his heart back on the right path. Normally when someone is in V-fib, they are pretty much dead. After they are shocked, even if their heart starts again, they are usually comatose for several days even if they survive. Not this guy. After every shock he would come around briefly and scream.

Pulling into the ER, I shocked him one last time. "Stop it, God damn it!" he yelled, and just then he puked all over the firefighter's boots, which I thought was funny because, like I already said, I don't like brownnosers.

Wheeling him into the emergency room, you could smell the burnt hair from all the shocks. I explained to the doc what was going on, and that I had shocked him several times. The doctor looked at me as if I was mentally challenged, and he said that I more than likely had a faulty monitor. He said, "It's highly unlikely that this patient has been in actual V-fib several times and is still talking."

After placing the patient on the hospital's monitor, he went into V-fib again and was shocked by the doctor himself. Once again the patient responded with colorful metaphors. At least, in the end, I felt some vindication. I only wish he would have puked on the doc. How dare he question *me*? I went to trade school.

As with this last patient, there are some who leave out a lot of important information that would really benefit them if they told us. I can't even give a rough estimate of how many patients I've transported to the emergency room that have left out the most important information, such as their history of cardiac problems, diabetes, or high blood pressure. Even though they told me they had no relevant medical history, when we arrive at the ER they suddenly become a wealth of information.

I will tell the nursing staff that even though the patient's blood pressure is elevated, they have stated they have no history of high blood pressure. Once I have given my report, the patient will tell the staff that he or she does, in fact, have a history of hypertension and that he's on previously unmentioned medications. This, needless to say, makes me look like an incompetent boob in front of the staff.

Sometimes the patients are their own worst enemies. This job would be perfect if not for the patients.

Chapter 17

Did you know that some people will call us because they have the misconception that by calling an ambulance, they will get evaluated more quickly in the emergency room? I don't know where this urban legend started, but if you call me for bullshit such as a toothache and use this excuse, you will end up in the back of the waiting room. The pure selfishness of this train of thought amazes me. The fact that some people will place their trivial complaints above all others' true emergencies is twisted.

I recently ran a call on an elderly woman who I've responded to several times over the years. Most of the time it was to help her back into bed after she'd fallen going to the toilet. Naturally, the calls always came after midnight, and this call was at three in the morning.

This woman is over 200 pounds, and for the most part, had been dead weight when lifting her up. This last time presented a different situation, however, as once again, her husband met us at the front door.

"We meet again!" said the husband with the same sheepish grin he always greeted us with. The first 10 or 20 times I ran calls at this address, I felt sorry for them—but not *this* time.

Entering through the front door, I found the woman standing with her walker. "What's the problem this time?" I asked.

"I've had trouble peeing for the last month, and my doctor said that if I didn't improve within a month's time, I should go to the hospital," she answered.

Trouble taking a piss! Yes, you read it right. That is why an ambulance was called to this residence, not for a sudden onset of illness. Like she said, it had been going on for a month, but for some reason at 3 a.m. that morning it became an emergency.

When I asked her why she had called an emergency ambulance—a vehicle, like I stated before, that equals a mobile emergency room—she said, "I know if we go by ambulance, we won't have to sit in the waiting room."

Being that no one, including the media, seems to care about this subject, I take it upon myself to enlighten people. I informed this last patient that because she felt too important to sit in a waiting room, she was preventing me from helping those in *real* need of emergency care.

I said, "Lady, because of your impatience, if one of your neighbors should suffer a heart attack, I can't help them, and they could possibly die."

"Well, I can't pee, and you're here now so just take me to the hospital," she replied.

Of course, I took her to the hospital. What the hell else could I do? She called and we hauled.

Why should I even give a shit? Nobody else does. I wish I could just do my 24 hours and not care. Unfortunately, I can't and I let it get to me when I should just turn a blind eye like everyone else. Maybe the reason I can't ignore it like some people is because I'm the one running on this bullshit at all hours of the night. The thoughts and views of the street medic have never been a priority with those at the top and I wonder if they ever will be. The higher echelon people get paid more than they deserve while taking credit for our actions and sleeping all night. They have proven to me that they have no integrity, so why would they ruin a good thing by listening to us.

Firefighters and police have what is called high-risk retirement, and recently EMS employees have been placed in that category. This means we can collect our benefits immediately after we retire instead of waiting until we reach our sixties.

When I first heard of high-risk, I thought it was because our job can at times be very dangerous, but that wasn't the reason. We are allowed to collect benefits early because our life expectancy is less than average. This is due to the fact the stress we work under, and the conditions we work in, make us more susceptible to medical problems such as hypertension and heart disease. Additionally, we encounter many other communicable diseases every shift.

Lately at my service there has been a lot of talk about getting us *ballistic* vests or bulletproof vests. A few years ago I had personally asked one of my former chiefs if we could have these types of vests because we respond to a variety of violent situations.

I was told *no*. He said that it wouldn't be cost-effective and it was our job to avoid potentially dangerous scenes. The big problem with that line of thought is that any scene can turn violent at any time, and you won't know until it's too late.

A co-worker of mine was actually stabbed in the back by an elderly woman with a pair of sewing shears. This was an old lady in a moo moo. Why would anyone think of her as potentially dangerous? You just never know.

Stage near the scene until law enforcement advises it is secure and safe—that is our procedure. The cops have vests and guns while we have nothing, and we are on the same scene. When I asked if we could have pepper spray or some other means of self-defense, that request was also shot down. I was told these means of self-defense could be a possible liability to the county.

So the EMS workers being injured or killed in an act of violence is acceptable because the powers that be are afraid our pepper spray might affect a bystander. Now that's twisted logic.

Michelle and I responded to a stabbing, and as we were en route, dispatch advised, "Law enforcement on scene. Scene secured."

Michelle was familiar with the address and told me she had run on our patient before and that he was an asshole. There were at least four cop cars on scene as we arrived, and a woman was being taken from the house in handcuffs. Entering the home, we found an elderly man sitting on a chair in the front room. He had stab wounds to both sides of his neck and was bleeding profusely.

We quickly moved him to our stretcher and began treating him while a handful of cops stood around watching. Michelle was right. This guy was an asshole and, even with his wounds, was giving us attitude. The woman in cuffs was his wife, and I guess she'd finally had enough of his crap and snapped. She had actually tried to poison him, but when that didn't work, she stabbed the shit out of him. It's on calls like this that I actually feel happy about being single.

Michelle was starting her second IV as I held pressure dressings on his wounds to slow the bleeding. Just then a door to a room behind us flew open, and an adult male who looked like Charles Manson came barging out.

"What the fuck is going on!" he demanded.

Our so-called police protection spun around and seemed more shocked than Michelle and I. This was the adult son of the patient and no one knew he was there. The cops had advised that the scene was secure, but had failed to clear the house room by room. You would think that would be standard operating procedure, but as I have tried to point out, nothing is standard on a call. This guy could have been armed. Even though the cops were somewhat protected with their vests, my partner and I were left with our asses in the breeze.

When you work this job long enough, you develop street smarts, and at times you can sense when a situation may escalate to violence. An example would be *not* wearing a stethoscope around your neck, as they often do in the movies, when dealing with a person who is emotionally disturbed. You know this person can freak out at any moment, and if he or she should grab both ends of the scope, you'll find yourself up close and personal with their face—and yes, they sometimes bite.

CHAPTER 18

Children always change the dynamic of a call, even if it's one where the child is in fact okay but the parents are not maintaining. Another partner and I were working one December day when we got a call for a six-year-old girl whose foot was stuck in her bike. The girl's mother was obviously upset and we tried to calm her down as we checked on the girl. Her foot was stuck between the bike's pedal and the frame. One of the fire departments had also responded to the call with us. There was no obvious injury, but the girl was scared and crying all the same.

At first we attempted to free her with soap and water but that didn't work. We soon realized the fire department would have to cut the bike apart to extricate her foot. When a hacksaw didn't work, the firefighters broke out a heavy duty circular saw and the kid really got scared. We told her that she would be all right, and as the fire crew cut the frame, I put my hand between her foot and the blade. I had run calls with this fire crew when they had to cut cars apart, and I knew they wouldn't cut me. I just thought shielding the kid from the blade with my hand might comfort her.

We were finally able to free the girl, but in doing so, her bike was destroyed. She was crying because her bike was ruined and also, I think, because a bunch of big ugly emergency workers scared her. My partner and I felt bad. This kid's family didn't have a lot of money and that bike was a big thing for her.

We talked about it as we were leaving the scene and decided to buy her a new bicycle. There just happened to be a store that sold bikes near the apartment complex we had just left. We went to the store and bought the girl a new bike.

The expression on the mom's face when we showed up at her door was priceless, and a very confused little girl seemed happy. I felt really good about that, it being the Christmas season and all.

A couple days later a local newspaper called me at home and said the story of this call was going to be printed. I agreed to answer a few questions after telling the reporter to never call me at home again.

When I'm on duty, it is fair game and I'll answer anything asked of me as long as my department approves. Off duty is a different story. I try not to even think about the job while on my own time, let alone answer some stranger's questions.

I gave the newspaper reporter a brief summary of the call and again asked them to respect my privacy. What had started out as a nice gesture was becoming another PR ploy by my department. Speaking only for myself, I didn't do it for EMS or fake recognition. I did it for a little kid who needed a bicycle.

When the article came out, I wasn't in the picture and I am proud of that. The kid was happy, I felt good about myself, and that was all I needed. That's more important than false accolades or a pat on the back.

Although there was no actual medical problem on the last call, it ended up being legitimate. It would be nice if everyone knew when and *when not* to call 911.

I remember channel surfing one time, and coming across a cartoon telling kids when to call 911. To this day I have yet to see anything in any medium advising adults when it is prudent to call for an ambulance. It really amazes me how stupid people can truly be. I've touched on some of the dumb stuff we run on but that's just the tip of the iceberg.

Following are some brief examples of why my truck couldn't respond to *real* calls due to stupidity:

1. Being called out at 2 a.m. to respond to a house to open an aspirin bottle.
2. Having a person call because they needed a ride to the pharmacy.

3. Showing up at a doctor's office for a patient already pronounced dead by the doctor.

4. Transporting someone who was involved in a minor MVC and denies injury because he thinks he *might* have an injury from it later—after he talks to a lawyer.

5. Someone calling because they think the sugar powder from their morning donut might be anthrax.

6. The lady who was able to tell dispatch she was choking on an ice cube.

7. Transporting a guy from the alcohol rehab center because he was drunk.

8. Picking up an old man with dementia from a nursing home because he keeps crawling in bed with the old ladies.

9. A person calling because he wants his blood sugar checked even though he feels fine and isn't diabetic, because he saw some medical show on TV.

10. Finally, my all-time favorite—responding to a home just because the occupant wanted to see if her brand new medical alarm worked.

I'll never understand how people like the ones in the previous examples *think*. I wish it was simply a matter of being ignorant, but I know some are so selfish and uncaring of their fellow man that they just don't give a shit. I can't stress enough the fact that if you call an ambulance for trivial bullshit, you can literally be aiding in someone's death. Unfortunately, when I explain this to some people, they show utter indifference. They just don't care. Needless to say, that is very disheartening and it really alters my outlook on humanity and where our society is headed.

I had this elderly man who had a major stroke while eating at a restaurant, and as we were trying to treat him, he began to vomit. I heard some lady at a table behind us complaining about her meal being ruined. This guy was dying and all she cared about was feeding her fat face.

The really messed-up thing is that people like her are the first to bitch about how important their loved ones are, and how we aren't doing enough. If a person doesn't care about their fellow man, why should I care about them?

I can't argue this, as it was my decision to take on this job. I treat and don't judge, at least not on scene—and it's hard for me to keep my mouth shut.

CHAPTER 19

Earlier I took some shots at Hollywood, but the truth is I could probably earn an Academy Award for my acting performance on the job. Regardless of how idiotic someone who called us might be, I can make it appear as though they are the most important person on the planet. My facial expressions and demeanor will have them totally convinced that I really give a shit, even though I obviously don't. If Stanley Kubrick was still alive, I could see him at least casting me in a cameo in my own life story.

You see, this job is a game, and the sooner you figure that out, the easier it is to play. When the newness of the job wears off, and you see the true reality of it, it's easier to accept the insanity. I try to explain this to newer medics but some just don't get it, and they make the job harder than it needs to be. An example would be ones who take information from dispatch and run with it. If they are told the patient is having a stroke, then that's all they see. I take the dispatch information with a grain of salt, and determine what is actually going on when I get on scene.

I sometimes wish dispatch would just give an address and let me figure out what's going on when I get there. I don't care if it's a plane full of nuns crashing into a busload of kids, I'll deal with the situation when I get there. You train yourself to deal with the unexpected.

After all these years there isn't much that surprises me anymore and I regret that. I used to love the feeling of responding to the unknown, but now everything is just another call. The novelty dissolves over time, and at least for me, every shift is like the movie *Ground Hog Day*. The same calls, only with different faces day in and day out.

Speaking of faces, it has gotten to the point where I can tell if a call is stupid or not, just by looking at the face of the person who called. I'm not sure if it's the eyes or just the expression, but for some reason I can sense stupidity. I guess it's a sense acquired over time. When I'm on a totally bogus scene, the caller always has the same clueless look on his or her face. It doesn't matter what ethnic background a person has, their look is always the same. Open your old high school yearbook, paying special attention to the dumbest looking faces. You'll understand the look I'm speaking of.

Drunks! I've mentioned only a few of my drunk-related calls. Because this is a major problem affecting EMS, I want to tell you about some of my most memorable ones.

I ran a call out in the eastern part of the county, another bad rural MVC. A mother and father were driving their young son home from school when they were hit head-on by a drunk driver. The parents were killed instantly and the boy was ejected. I was the second unit on scene and was given the drunk because the first unit, naturally, took the child.

Moving past my brothers, who were working on the boy, I made my way to my patient who was entrapped in what was left of his vehicle. The dash had crushed in around him and his legs were grossly entangled. He was semi-conscious and smelled of booze. Empty beer cans cluttered the front floorboard, and he was begging for help. At no time did my patient express any concern for the people he hit.

"Don't let me die!" is all he kept saying.

What a selfish piece of shit, I thought to myself. This asshole had just orphaned a kid and he didn't even care.

Ignoring my own feelings, I concentrated on saving this guy. Both of his legs were mangled and he was going into shock. I told the firefighters who were trying to extricate him that he wasn't going to make it if they didn't get him out quick.

"If we yank him out, it looks like one of his legs might rip off," a firefighter said.

I replied, "Fuck his leg! If I can't secure his airway and start an IV, he will die."

They finally got him out and both of his legs were only held on by tendons. After securing him to a backboard, I started two IV's so I could give him fluid to stabilize his blood pressure.

With the IV's established, I prepared for a RSI (Rapid Sequence Intubation). While my partner pushed the paralytics into the IV, I leaned down next to the patient's ear, and I told him we were giving him meds so I could place an airway tube and breathe for him.

As the medications took effect I whispered in his ear. "I hope you can hear me because I want you to know you just killed two people." Even paralyzed, I could tell by his eyes he had heard me.

He ended up losing both legs which I thought was poetic justice, as the boy had lost both parents. I can only hope he has nightmares until he dies.

As someone who drinks too much myself, I kind of feel like a hypocrite bashing drunks I've run on, but then again, I've never been so drunk as to get behind the wheel and endanger innocents. I just can't understand how some people can do that. I personally think if a drunk kills somebody, they should be forced to watch the autopsy of their victim. Maybe then they'll realize what they have done.

I've run on numerous people who have had multiple DUI's, and they're still allowed to drive.

Maybe the judges who set these people loose on society should also be in on the autopsy.

Last year I had to testify at the trial of a man I had done a blood draw on after he had killed two people while driving drunk. His van hit a motorcycle killing both riders. This guy had ten previous DUI's, and yet he was allowed to be on the road.

At no time did he show any remorse, and in fact, he tried to say his female passenger was driving. What a piece of shit. I felt like Jack Nicholson in *A Few Good Men* as I sat on the witness stand. I stared right at the son of a bitch as I testified, and I can't describe how good it felt. I shot down everything the defense threw at me.

When the district attorney told me my testimony helped get the guy 20 years in prison, I felt as though I had given out some justice for all the DUI victims I had run on over the years. My day in court was for them.

I must admit, some drunk calls are just downright funny. Some years ago we were called for a guy passed out behind a bar. This guy was so hammered that I had to use ammonia inhalants to wake him up. He didn't like that, and came up swinging.

He was a big guy and normally I would have been worried, but he was so trashed that every time he swung at us, he spun around like a top and fell down. In fact, it was so entertaining to watch, I started egging him on.

"Get up you big puss," I said between laughs. "You can do better than that."

After four or five swings and falls, he suddenly transformed into a ninja and tried to kick us. I was laughing so hard I almost pissed myself when a police officer arrived and ended the fun. Drunks hurting themselves are victimless crimes in my eyes, so I get a lot of satisfaction from it.

There was another call behind a bar in which the outcome was a little different. Like the last one, it came in as a drunk passed out. Arriving on scene, a female bartender met us in the back parking lot. It was about 3 a.m. and cold as hell outside. I asked her what was going on. She pointed to a car in the poorly-lit parking lot.

"It's Buddy. He's a regular and he got really drunk tonight so we kicked him out."

Walking up to the car, I found the driver lying back in the driver seat. "Wake up Buddy!" I said as I shook him. No response. *This guy must be bombed*, I thought, as I told my partner to get some ammonia and a flashlight.

Shining the flashlight into the car, it was obvious I wouldn't need the ammonia. Buddy was still holding the large caliber revolver he had placed under his chin. As I shined the light up, I noticed the back of his head splattered all over the roof of the car.

Well Buddy, at least you did it right, I thought to myself.

"When he wakes up, tell him he is no longer welcome here," I heard the bartender say from behind me.

"I think he got that point," I replied.

136 TONES

Chapter 20

We run hundreds of calls for suicide attempts where someone is just looking for attention. I have had people cut their wrists with disposable razors, and some try to overdose on laxatives. What the hell?

As someone who lost a loved one to suicide, calls like these really piss me off. I have more respect for the people like Buddy. I hate to see anyone kill themselves, but if you're going to do it, do it. Don't fuck around and tie up my ambulance with selfish attention-getting bullshit.

I know it sounds callous, but try to see it from my point of view. While I'm dealing with the girl who took five Tylenol pills, who's saying she wants to kill herself because her man screwed her sister, someone else is having a real emergency.

I've mentioned the selfishness of our society several times already, but I can't stress it enough. Get over yourselves! Don't look at EMS as a "catch all"—because we have our own problems.

I once saw a commercial on TV talking about Post Traumatic Stress Disorder (PTSD) and its signs and symptoms. It gave 11 examples, of which I had seven. When I hear people whining about trivial bullshit, I could give a damn.

Even though we are the least paid in the medical food chain, we are expected to be psych experts, cardiologists, pulmonologists, general practitioners, and OB/GYNs, all the while not being given any sympathy or compassion by administration. I actually had a captain bitch me out because a family member of one of my patients said I scratched a wall with my stretcher. The fact that the patient was in cardiac arrest, and I saved his life, didn't seem to matter.

In the long run, letting stuff like that stress me out is my own fault. I didn't get into this line of work expecting any thank yous, but having unappreciative assholes and an administration that always sides against us is a real bummer. The mental trauma of dealing with life's most painful and graphic situations is secondary.

Recently I ran a call where two gay lovers got in a fight and one was stuck in the arm with a fork. When I arrived, the cops told me the *forker* had left the scene and the victim was in the house yelling profanities. Always dutiful, I approached the house and asked the man inside if he needed assistance.

"Come inside—and I'll shoot you!" was his reply.

I informed dispatch that the man had just threatened to shoot us, and we were leaving the scene. Moments later, one of my supervisors arrived and said this. "If you don't know if he has the means to shoot you, then he should be evaluated." Translation—you should let him shoot you and then refuse to treat him.

My service is so afraid of being sued by even made-up reasons that sometimes it feels as though they are willing to sacrifice us. I know that's not the case, but sometimes it feels that way. Maybe it's just me, but that in itself is a stressor.

Common sense—it really boggles my mind how so much of our population is lacking it. I have too many examples of this to mention them all, but I'll try to give some good ones. We run on a lot of diabetic patients, mostly for hypoglycemia or low blood sugar. I've had patients who have been diabetic for years and take insulin without eating afterwards. When this happens, a person's sugar can drop very low. By the time I get to them, they are usually unresponsive.

The treatment for this is to administer sugar via IV, and as the patient's sugar rises, they become responsive. My first question for the patients usually involves asking them if they ate after taking their insulin.

"I wasn't hungry," is the typical reply. Even though they know their sugar will drop without eating, they do it anyway. I've never understood that. Why would someone knowingly do that to themselves?

Some people are their own worst enemies. Although they're a pain in the ass, they do keep food on my table. Has the thought of sticking your hand under a running lawnmower ever crossed your mind? Not mine either, but it made for an interesting call.

Even when I'm off duty I see potential patients. The other day I saw a lady driving down the road talking on a cell phone while simultaneously fixing her hair in the mirror. I wondered how her hair would look if she ran head-on into a telephone pole.

Speaking of head-on, I almost lost two of my brothers last week when their unit was hit almost head-on by a pickup. They were responding to a call when a careless driver blew past other vehicles that had yielded for the ambulance. The unit was totaled as was the pickup that hit them. One of the crew had to be extricated and flown to a trauma center. I didn't respond to this call as it was on the opposite side of the county.

For my brothers and sisters who did respond, it was very traumatizing. It is one thing to respond to a stranger, but when you see your co-workers hurt, it's very disturbing. I know from personal experience, as I responded to a similar call some years ago. My hands were literally shaking as I tried to help my injured comrades. Fortunately both my friends on this recent call recovered from the injuries and concussions they received.

I had one of my own trucks creamed once. It was Easter morning 1995, and my partner and I were responding to a call. We stopped at an intersection and waited for all the traffic to yield before slowly proceeding across. Unfortunately, an old lady in a big-assed Buick didn't notice our lights and sirens. I was driving and caught her out of the corner of my eye just before impact. My partner damned near ended up in my lap.

The entire right front of the truck was destroyed, and even though we were both stunned, we immediately checked on the lady. Other than being shaken up, she was okay, so we moved both vehicles into a fast food parking lot and waited for our supervisor.

While we waited, my partner went and got us a couple sodas. When involved in an on-duty accident, a supervisor will respond with all kinds of paperwork to fill out. The one who came to this call was a real jerk that I can honestly say is the person I have despised more than anyone else in my life.

I was sitting on what was left of my hood when he arrived, and at no time did he show any concern for my partner or me. He asked us what had happened, and I explained what went down.

"There had to be some way you could have avoided this," he said in his typical condescending way.

"You are absolutely right, sir," I replied. "This could have been avoided if we didn't respond to the call in the first place."

He didn't like my answer, which was the point of it, so he started giving me shit because I didn't seem to be taking the situation seriously.

"You don't appear to be very upset about this," he said.

I wasn't. "It's called acceptance," I told him. "I've gone through the denial phase and now I accept the fact that some old bat smashed my truck."

That really pissed him off, which was very satisfying to me. I went even further and told him that if he wanted, I would lie on the ground and have a conniption fit, which again pissed him off.

This same piece of shit had told my partner and me we couldn't wear black tape on our badges after my girl killed herself. "We don't celebrate suicides," he told us. Needless to say, I can't stand the son of a bitch—and yes, he's still around. I look at it like he is the Lex Luthor to my Superman.

This has been a bad week for me and my brothers and sisters in our service. Not only have we received no pay raises in four years while our department heads and commissioners *have*, but we now have to pay for our insurance out of our own pockets.

Now, I know times are tough for everyone, but unless your job deals with making life and death decisions while putting your own life on the line, don't feel too bad. As I mentioned earlier, we've been told we do not deserve protective body armor, even though we are exposed to the same violence as law enforcement.

We have HazMat (Hazardous Materials) suits that none of us will ever wear, but they aren't bullet resistant. We are told that we'll be thankful we have them if there's another terrorist attack on our country.

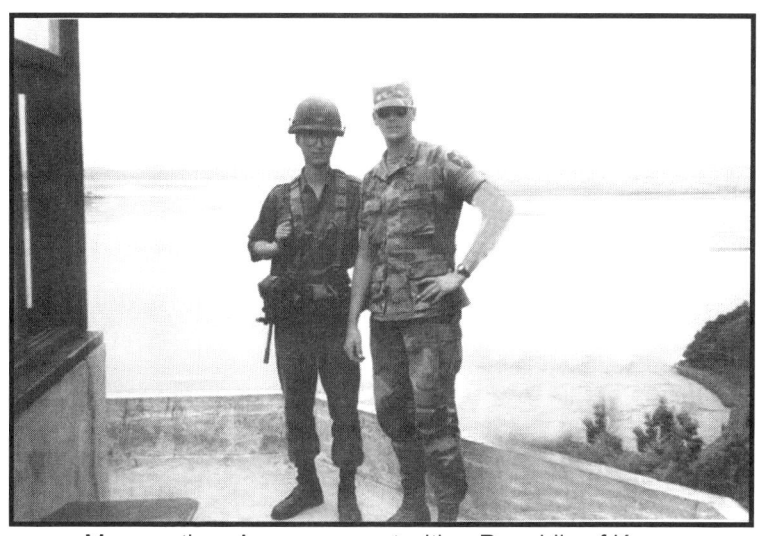

Me as a then Army sergeant with a Republic of Korea (ROK) soldier on DMZ during a tour of duty in Korea.

What has been the most effective weapon for our enemy? IEDs (Improvised Explosive Devices)—and it's only a matter of time before they use them against us in our country. Buy a trace-free cell phone from a convenience store and some fertilizer and other components, and you have a bomb. Even a computer-challenged person like me can figure that out.

Unfortunately, the powers that be don't see the forest for the trees and won't make any changes until one of us is dead. The average person sits at home and doesn't think about stuff like this, and that's the way it should be. Part of the reason we do what we do is because the majority of folks can't stomach it and don't want to accept some of the shit we deal with.

It's like serving in the Army. Every soldier does what he or she does to keep some form of normalcy in this world for the rest of us.

I speak of leadership, having some experience and background in it. I was a soldier for almost three years when I was promoted to sergeant. Before you can make that rank, you have to prove yourself as a person with leadership potential. There is a point system which includes performance evaluations, weapons qualifications, and experience. You must also graduate from one of the Army's leadership academies, which I did.

Don't get me wrong. In my service I do have some very fine supervisors, whom I really respect. It's just that having been a non-commissioned officer in the Army and having led soldiers in difficult situations, I find it hard to take some of these people seriously. I have integrity, and that is a big thing with me.

Forget the Webster's version. My version of integrity is—*I won't expect you to do something I wouldn't or haven't done myself.* When I was a sergeant, I always put my soldiers' welfare before my own. I learned from braver men than I that if you lead by example, your people will follow.

CHAPTER 21

Once again I must apologize for getting off track. I'm trying to give a true, honest example of life as a medic and I'm letting current and personal bullshit get in the way. For people who are reading this for more than entertainment, but as insight into a possible career move, I'll leave my last rant in.

If you become a paramedic, you'll get the uniform, the badge, and a lot of the previously mentioned bullshit regardless of which service you work for. That's just reality. You'll also get the satisfaction that comes from helping people who are truly in need. That's what has kept me going or else I would have hung it up a long time ago.

I just got off the phone with my old partner Jackie, and at the end of our conversation, she wished me a good day. That got me thinking. What is a *good day*?

Maybe if your kid got a good report card or the people in the office got you a cheesy birthday gift—

that's a good day to you. To me, a good day is when my partner and I survive another shift without being hurt or killed. An even better day is when I can say at the end of a shift that no one died. Nobody died! What a concept.

I know it must be hard for people not involved in emergency care to comprehend. I'm certainly not trying to belittle anyone, but seriously, can *everyone* say that? I had a good day because nobody died! That's a hell of a statement, and one I've made several times. That's it for my *soap boxing,* I promise. Be advised, though, I have broken many promises before.

I've mentioned some of my co-workers, but I need to delve further into this subject. My brother and sister EMS workers come from almost every walk of life. There are some who have multiple college degrees and some with GEDs. We have single moms who spent their last dime to attend EMT school, hoping for a better future for their kids, and people who were bound for med school but wanted to get a taste of the real world before making that commitment involving the next decade of their lives.

It doesn't matter where you come from. Like the military, when you all wear the same uniform and deal with the same hardships, you are family. It is a brotherhood.

Some of the folks I've worked with over the years are hard to describe. There was a guy who worked here for a while who was a complete asshole. When I say asshole, I mean absolutely everyone hated working with this guy. He was on a complete ego trip, which wouldn't have bothered me except he sucked as a paramedic. I would see him bitching out his EMT partners or firefighters, and I would tell him *to shut the fuck up*. Not to mention, off duty he was a nudist, and I would always find him talking about that at work.

Shortly before he left, he became a Christian fanatic, which in itself was a trip. He would sit on his bunk reading the Bible, and if the tones went off, he would typically react by saying *God damn it!*—while throwing the Bible down.

What a dick. Last I heard he started a cult or some such bullshit. I don't foresee another Waco incident; I mean *really*, where would Christian nudists hide their weapons? Sorry, that was in poor taste.

We also had a co-worker who was convinced she had been abducted by aliens. If you talked to her, that actually wasn't hard to believe. She was a nice girl, but really spacey—no pun intended.

148 TONES

CHAPTER 22

I've mentioned how some of my closest friends are EMS workers, and one of my best was James, to whom I dedicated this book.

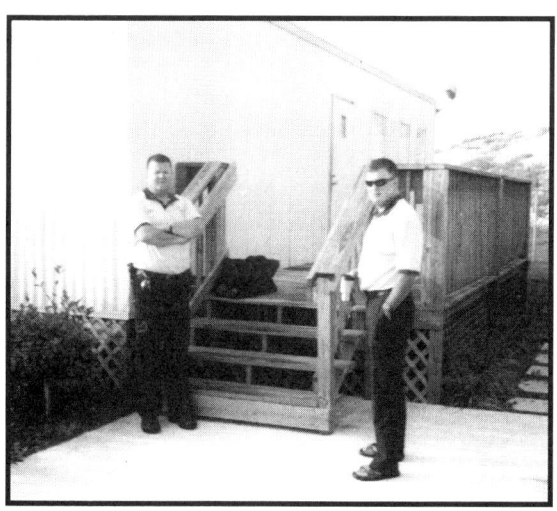

James, a true inspiration and his partner and my friend Jason.

I met James early in my career, as he was one of my instructors in both the EMT and paramedic programs. You could sense that a lot of the instructors were just there for the extra money from teaching because their regular pay sucked so badly. They didn't really care if their students were actually learning.

Not James. His heart was really in it, and he would stay after class to help students who were falling behind. The epitome of a paramedic, he seriously loved the job and helping strangers.

When I started with EMS, we worked together several times and developed a strong bond. Eventually we were on the same station rotation and I would see him every third day as my relief. As time went by, it amazed me how he never got burned out or let the bullshit get him down. He was an awesome husband, father, and friend. James and his wife even took in foster kids and treated them as if they were their own.

Whenever I had a bad call, such as a child I couldn't save, I could always talk to James. A few years ago he started having pain in his upper leg, which he initially thought was wear and tear from the job. He saw a doctor about it and that's when the bomb was dropped. James had bone cancer, and his family and friends were devastated.

He had surgery which involved replacing his femur with a metal rod. He was so strong that he was up walking in physical therapy within a few days. It seems just like yesterday his nurse caught me sneaking cheeseburgers into his room and chewed me out. I had to convince her that I was on my lunch break and the food was for me. After she stepped out, James and I laughed as he ate the burgers he had been craving.

While James was recovering, and on days he was off chemotherapy, I would gather our closest friends from EMS and visit him. We would bring food for his family and hang out with him. I think it was more for us than for him. We all loved him so much and had to let him know he wasn't forgotten.

If you have had a loved one suffer from cancer, you already know how cruel and unfair it is, and it didn't let up on James. For a brief period we thought it was gone because James had gone into remission, but like the true bitch it is, it came back with a vengeance.

James and the family moved to Georgia to try more aggressive treatment, but that ended up being futile as the cancer spread into his lungs. I drove up to see James with his old partner Jason, who truly was like a brother to him. Due to our work schedules, we could only spend two days, and they were the most important two days in my life to this point. Walking into his house, I almost broke down as I saw my friend lying in a hospital-type bed in the living room.

My friend and brother who had been so full of life and who had helped and saved so many, was nearing the end of his. He was so weak that there were only a few hours a day we could talk to him. We sat at his bedside and tried to make him more comfortable. We would adjust his pillows, get him water, and help him sit up to urinate. Even though he was in more pain than anyone should ever bare, he did not complain once. He wanted to be strong for his family and he was. I've met some brave people in my life but James was the bravest, and he will always be a hero to me.

On the morning we were leaving, we got up around 7 a.m. Because of his pain medications, James normally slept till ten, but he was awake when we got up. He stopped taking his pain meds so he would be awake to say good-bye. My God, when you think about it, it's beautiful. Someone loved his friends so much he let himself suffer unspeakable pain so he could say good-bye. I wish I could be that strong.

I leaned over his bed and gave him a hug and kissed his forehead. "I love you, Bro," I said as my eyes welled up.

"I love you too, Dave," he replied softly.

Those were the last words I heard from James, and I will cherish them for the rest of my life. He died two weeks later and was given a memorial service with full honors. EMS workers, nurses, firefighters, and law enforcement from several counties attended. There wasn't a dry eye in the place, especially when they did the last call for James.

God bless you, James. We will never forget. I miss you, my friend.

CHAPTER 23

Personal situations like the one just mentioned make it extremely hard to deal with the petty, selfish bullshit we see on a daily basis. But as usual, we have to suck up each situation regardless how trivial, and drive on.

I try to explain to newer EMT's and medics that people don't care about us until they need us, and even then, many times they treat us like shit. We have to at least portray ourselves as caring and concerned professionals. I guess that's the old soldier in me. You have to pump up and motivate the troops. Motivation—sometimes it's hard to maintain or even achieve depending on the call.

I had my first *geriatric loss of saliva and vaginal secretion* call the other day, and boy was my adrenalin pumping. The call came in as breathing problems, and when we knocked on the door, the man of the house answered.

"We're almost ready!" he said, closing the door.

My partner and I stepped back and looked at each other. Our expressions must have been the same because we didn't say a word. After two or three minutes I knocked again and entered the home.

I found the man and his wife in the front bedroom packing her bags. The couple, in their eighties, was discussing which housecoat the wife should wear. I asked who was having the breathing problem. The woman looked at me and said she could only breathe through her mouth because she took a new medication two days ago.

"I have lost all of my saliva and vaginal secretions," she explained.

Left speechless, and quickly realizing our patient was *batshit crazy,* we put her and her luggage on the stretcher, and took her to the hospital. Is that a motivating and inspirational call or what? I love my job.

I used to get really upset about the stupid calls until I realized they are kind of a godsend. When I'm dealing with some dipshit, there is no stress. So honestly, why should I care? As long as there isn't a more serious call I'm being kept from, who gives a shit? I know I have told you about my aggravations, but I am realizing it's not worth fighting a losing cause. In the past when I would inform some of my dumber callers of their ignorance, now I just load them up and transport. Nobody else cares, so why should I?

I wish all of what I just wrote was true, and then my story would be finished, but it's not. Although I do transport more of the bullshit than I used to without arguing, I still do care, and I still have more to tell. Let me get back to some of my more interesting calls. I've mentioned some of the Christmas calls I've run and even one on Easter, but I forgot to mention an actual Thanksgiving call. Well, I have one of those too.

It was actually about 2 a.m. in the morning, the day after Thanksgiving. My unit and another were at the motor pool after running an MVC together. There is an industrial facility next to the motor pool with train tracks running between them. After fueling our trucks, both of our units were returning to quarters. Just as both trucks pulled out of the motor pool, our headlights shined on what was left of an old pickup that had slammed into the side of a moving train.

We must have all been in some sort of shock at what we were viewing, because it took us a few seconds to react. The train was moving slowly, and the truck was bouncing as each train car brushed up against it. We told dispatch what we had just driven up on, and all four crew members gloved up and approached the wreckage.

On this call, I had only been on the job a little over a year and was the rookie among this group. This meant I was the only one who put on a protective helmet and jacket. (Quick note, these jackets, which we still use today are highly flammable. I could say something derogatory here, but I'll be good.)

Because my dumb ass was the only one to put on the gear, I was elected to climb in what was left of the truck and check the driver. This guy was so fucked. The engine was partially inside the cab, and he had agonal respirations (shallow and labored breathing). With the remnants of the truck still bouncing, I climbed in and checked him for a carotid pulse. Unbelievably, he had one. We had managed to pull him out just as the fire department arrived, and it was at this point we realized how messed up he was.

His legs were shattered and he had massive head and chest trauma. Before we could initiate care, he coded. Because I was still considered the new guy amongst my peers, they let me do all of the ALS (Advance Life Support) stuff. While still next to the truck, I intubated him, and once we were in the back of the unit, I did my first chest decompression.

This procedure involves sticking a large needle between the patient's ribs and into the chest because a lung is leaking air into the chest cavity causing it to collapse. When the needle pierces the chest cavity, it allows any air leaked into it from the affected lung to escape. This, in turn, allows the lung to fill with air.

By the time we got this guy to the ER, he was deader than dead, but at least he didn't go in vain, as I got to perform one of our more aggressive skills on a real person and not a training dummy. I did something some medics with 20 years in had never done.

Fifty or so decompressions later, it's hard to believe I was actually nervous about that first one. I was even given a pretty cool nickname a while ago by my co-workers—Trauma Dave. I had a bad stretch of serious trauma calls one year and the title was given to me. There was one week during that year where I had six trauma alerts, did two decompressions, one chricothyrotomy, two RSIs, and had four fatalities. I guess I earned that moniker.

In fact, I've actually had photos taken of me in action printed in *JEMS* magazine. That's the *Journal of Emergency Medicine.* Although I never read it anymore, at that time being featured in it was a big deal in the emergency world.

I had friends from all over the state say how cool it was seeing photos of me in it, and that was an awesome feeling. My service never said anything, which was no surprise. Getting positive vibes from my peers means more to me than anything coming down from the ivory tower, because they have walked the walk.

Trauma! That is what most people think of when it comes to EMS. I can't tell you how many times I've been asked by non-emergency folk for the gory details. Too many movies—remember the Hollywood thing I mentioned.

In this job you will eventually be introduced to the gore. Not everyone is going to see it as early as I did in my career. In fact, a medic will probably run a couple hundred calls for each good trauma call. Man, just saying that sounds weird—*good* trauma call. How can any trauma call be *good*? We get so bored with the mundane, that some of us actually wish for a major trauma call. Unfortunately, sometimes our wishes come true, and then we regret it because we suddenly remember how much work and stress can be involved while working a bad one.

Medical calls can be exciting also, but there's no comparison to pulling up on a major trauma scene. Working a cardiac arrest, stroke, or severe respiratory call can get the adrenalin pumping, but those calls don't compare to a critical shooting, stabbing, or MVC. The graphic visions on these calls can drastically change the tone of a scene. Working on someone entrapped in a mangled vehicle flipped over on the interstate is a little more exciting than arriving at a shuffleboard court or mobile home. Naturally, your concern for the patient is the same regardless of what environment they are found in.

There was a paramedic student that I precepted (mentored) a while ago who couldn't wait to run a bad call. Medic students ride ten shifts with a real medic crew near the end of their program. This gives them a chance to learn about the real world as well as be evaluated by someone other than the instructors they had in the classroom.

Because some medics who precept students are on a total power trip and dog the student, I've always tried to take it easy on them. A lot of the students have some emergency background and may already be working somewhere as an EMT. The rest have very little street experience like the student I'm writing about here.

This kid was really gung ho and couldn't wait to see a bad call. During his first eight or nine shifts, he didn't get to see much. All the calls we were running were pretty routine, and my student was getting discouraged.

"I wish we would get something good," he said. "I spent all that time in class and haven't had one decent call since I started my ride time."

I told him to be careful what he wished for and that the real calls would eventually come. In this job you can't let your guard down. You may go months without a serious call, and if you get too comfortable, it will come back to bite you.

On one of his last shifts with me, my student finally got his wish. We had two fatality vehicle accidents and a cardiac arrest. During the first shifts he asked me how I deal with running so many routine calls, and I told him it comes with the job. At the end of the last shift he asked how I deal with so many critical calls, and I gave him the same answer. It's the job. Like I mentioned at the beginning of my story, it's not anything like it's portrayed in the movies.

Another cool thing about the job has to do with the sights you get to see, and I don't mean in a carnage kind of way. I have been in multimillion dollar homes and dwellings that are in worse shape than your neighbor's lawn shed. We get to see places in our community that most didn't know existed.

There was this home I was in that had four levels, an elevated five-car garage, and a bar that looked like it came right out of Vegas. We were called for a cardiac arrest and found the owner DOA on the floor of the largest bedroom I had ever seen. It was on the upper level and had a circular balcony overlooking the bay. There was a projection screen TV, mini-bar, kitchen, and a gigantic bathroom with a Jacuzzi. While my partner stayed with the wife and got info, I carried our kits downstairs.

I could have taken the elevator, but I wanted to soak up each and every level. On the second to last level I stopped and stood in awe as I looked at the frosted glass doors at the entrance to the main bar. Setting the kits down, I slowly opened the doors, and for a brief moment, I had found Nirvana.

There were two eight-foot pool tables in the center of the room with the fanciest pool lights I have ever seen. On the right was a full bar that could have substituted for the one in *Cheers*. It had half a dozen beer taps and a large flat screen behind it. On the left there was an Elvis pinball machine and four or five slot machines. I realized at that very moment how much I really should have paid attention in school, or maybe studied acting.

I was so awed, it took me a second to realize a friend of the dead guy had shown up, and she was asking me what was going on. Changing my expression from one of complete envy to one of remorse, I told her what happened and she took the elevator upstairs.

It was a shame the owner had died, but damn if the man didn't have a good life while it lasted. In the end, that's all that counts. I know in some eyes material things shouldn't really matter, but being as I have never had those things, they make me want them.

Money can't buy you happiness. What idiot came up with that saying? It may not buy me happiness, but I'm sure I would suffer through it.

On the other end of the spectrum I have been in some real shitholes that actually made me feel rich, if only for a brief moment. I remember a call we had in a house that was so old and decrepit we thought it might cave in on us. Old weathered and rotting wood was the only thing holding up the rusted tin roof. We were called there for an elderly woman who was having breathing problems, and naturally, she was in the back bedroom. She had probably lived there her whole life and it was night time when we got the call.

The only light in the place was in her back room. As we entered the house, the rotted floor boards were cracking under our feet and the smell of cat piss filled the air. I had only taken two or three steps when my foot went through the floor.

"Be careful!" the old woman yelled from the back room.

This house was about a hundred years old and I was up to my knee in floor. Not wanting to cut my leg on a jagged piece of wood, I asked my partner to shine a light at the hole in the floor. As the light shined down, I felt something on my boot, and as I looked down, I saw a rat the size of a football sitting on it. I screamed like a little girl as I fell back out of the hole, which my partner on this call found very amusing. With one obstacle down, we followed the light to our patient. I guess you could say she was a bit of a pack rat because we had to climb over cardboard boxes and piles of old musty clothes just to reach her room.

    Entering the room, my back suddenly started to ache as we finally laid eyes on the body behind the voice that had called us for help. If you've seen the movie *Return of the Jedi*, that should help give you a good visual. Does Jabba the Hutt ring a bell? This poor thing weighed about 500 pounds, and she was wedged between her bed and the dresser.

    America's heroes, the fire department, had to come to the rescue, and it took six of us to get her out and into the truck. The situation and conditions she was living in were really sad, and I would never have known places like that were in my town if not for this job. Even sadder is the fact that her place is just one of many. Like my mom, who has been the strongest and most influential person in my life, has always told me: "We should count our blessings," and "There, but for the grace of God go I."

Chapter 24

At times when I'm really feeling sorry for myself, all I have to do is think about some of the truly needy and desperate people I've run calls on. Some can barely afford to buy food and it makes me see that being a little late on a car payment isn't that bad.

Just this last Thanksgiving, Angie and I ran on a woman who lived with her adult daughter. The daughter had called because her mother had been getting progressively weaker over the last few days. The house was in disarray, and the daughter told us they had not eaten in almost a week because she had lost her job.

They were both very embarrassed for having called us, and as I talked to the mom, she said she didn't want to go to the hospital because she thought we had people worse off than her to treat. That is a rare thing to see in this job, a person who actually cares about others more than herself. After we checked her vital signs and she signed a release saying she was refusing transport, we left.

Feeling very humbled, Angie and I drove to the nearest grocery store and bought them some food and bottled water. Bread, peanut butter and jelly, and because they didn't have turkey at the store, we got them fried chicken. We figured that because of the fact it was Thanksgiving and all, they should have some sort of bird to eat.

When we returned with the food, they both began crying and hugging us. "God bless you!" they kept saying, and we wished them a Happy Thanksgiving. Driving back to the station, Angie and I didn't say a word, but I know for that brief moment in time we felt some personal satisfaction. There, but for the grace of God.

Speaking of Angie, my administration was hesitant about letting us partner up because of our poor attitudes. In our service, pointing out the shortcomings is considered having a *bad attitude*. It amazes me how some people just roll over and accept the fact that they are not being treated fairly.

God only knows why that is—and after reading this book so far, you might find it hard to fathom, but God is someone I deeply believe in. What I find hard to believe is how some people use God to justify things.

"It's God's will." That is a saying I don't really understand. I've heard family members say it was God's will when one of their loved ones had died. This bugs me, especially when the death was not a pleasant one, like a bad car wreck. I can't believe that God wills anyone to die. I look at it like this—whatever happens was going to happen, and it's how you lived your life that determines where your soul ends up. I prefer the saying "It's out of God's hands."

There are many times I wish the Almighty would intervene, though, like suddenly making the more ignorant 9-11 callers smart. Man that would be a dream comes true, because our call load would plummet. What a concept, people calling 9-11 only for *real* emergencies. That really is hard to imagine. If that was the case, I couldn't complain about my pay anymore, because I would only be running about one call a shift.

Speaking of folks calling the now-famous, or should I say *infamous* emergency number, the job was so much easier before cell phones. When I first started with EMS, cell phones were still relatively new. Now that everyone from geriatrics to five-year-olds has one, the calls are never-ending. I think some folks call 9-11 just so they can say they called 9-11.

Interstate calls are the worst. Someone will see the blur of a car on the side of the road as they blow by doing 80 and grab the trusty cell phone. It had to be an accident, right? I mean, why would somebody just stop on the side of a busy highway? I guess the thought of people stopping to rest or read a map never comes to mind.

Sadly, there are some interstate highway calls that end up being very legit and the phone calls more than justified. On one dark and drizzling night ... Wait a minute! Stop! I know what you're thinking. This guy is either trying to eat, or it is a dark and drizzling night *whenever* he gets a call.

What the hell! I'm sorry but these stories and weather conditions are true. Now back to this call. A family from New York was on the way to their grandparents who lived south of my county. They had pulled over on the shoulder of the road to secure some luggage that was coming loose on the roof of their minivan. Meanwhile, an overloaded semi-tractor trailer was driving recklessly down the interstate, swerving between lanes. The driver of a full-size pickup truck tried to get by the semi and was struck in the rear end, sending it careening off the road on a collision course with the van.

As the mom and dad stood at the rear of the vehicle strapping down the loose bags, the pickup slammed into them. The mom was thrown about 50 feet and was killed instantly. Her husband had been thrown to the side after the impact. One of his legs was partially amputated after being pinched between the bumpers.

My partner and I were the first of three units to arrive. Approaching the van, I vaguely remember two little girls standing amongst some bystanders.

"Please help my family," the father pleaded with us.

My partner and some firefighters who had arrived after us began treating the father while I went to the mother. She looked like a broken doll. She was on her back, but her head was face down in the dirt. Even though she was obviously dead, I knelt down and turned her head face up. To this day I have no idea why I did that.

I returned to the crash scene to check on other patients and to help my partner. A firefighter who was now with the little girls said they had been in the van but were unharmed. If I had to guess, I would say they were approximately ages eight and ten.

I went to work helping my partner with the dad who was now delirious from shock. We had managed to stop the bleeding and established two IV's that were running wide open to replace the fluid he had lost. The faint sound of a medivac helicopter was in the distance when I realized that there was the voice of a small child coming from behind me.

"How come nobody's helping my mommy?" I heard her cry. I suddenly felt as if I had been punched in the gut. Those words and this call would haunt me for a long time. I couldn't bring myself to look at the kids after it was over. I read in the paper the next day that the mother of the woman killed had died in a wreck when she was a child. I can only hope those little girls don't carry on that legacy.

Chapter 25

Well, that was a very depressing recollection and now I think some levity is needed. So please, allow me to reflect upon another tale. I know it will be hard to accept as truth, but once again, it happened exactly how I remember.

Before I begin this one, for the record, I should mention a recent study suggests that all memories are distorted. Again, this is something I neither created nor researched, but it was done by some very educated people.

You know the type—the people we used to laugh at for studying while we were slacking off. Yes, those people, the ones running the world now.

Anyway, some of them researched a group of individual's memories and compared them to the actual events involving the subjects. Some had left out important elements, while others embellished. So, regarding my next recollection, I will just say that I was ripped and had a six pack of abs. That was a joke by the way.

I was working one day with a very good paramedic partner. He was a little too by the book for me sometimes, but excellent at the job none the less. We got a call for a shooting downtown, not far from our station. Pulling up to the scene, we saw a young man sitting on the curb. The city police were already there, and I asked them where the patient was. They pointed to the guy on the curb. This call happened around midnight, so I asked one of the cops to shine his flashlight on the dude.

To my amazement, not only had the guy been shot, but the bullet hit him right in the middle of his forehead. It obviously had been a small caliber bullet, I'm guessing a 25. After hitting his skull, the bullet had ridden under the scalp, gone over the top of his head, and finally, exited in the back of his head.

It was a very strange sight to see. This young man, maybe 20, had been shot point blank in the face and he was talking to me.

"What happened bro?" I asked, as if it wasn't self-evident.

"That mutha-fucka stole my crack and shot me in the head!" he exclaimed.

My partner was not too pleased when he saw me walk the patient to the truck. Normally someone with this type of wound would be secured to a backboard before being moved, so as to avoid any possible spinal injury.

I didn't give a shit though, as the patient stood up and headed toward the truck before I could stop him. This dickbag was more concerned about the crack he'd had stolen from him than anything else. He would have sold that shit to school kids if it would have made him any money, so using his own vernacular, fucka him.

This last partner and I ran more than a few interesting calls together. Another one that sticks out in my mind was a cardiac arrest we had. This big fat guy dropped on his kitchen floor and we started working on him with a couple firefighters helping us. While the firefighters performed CPR, my partner was at the head preparing to intubate.

I was at the patient's side trying to start an IV, when all of a sudden I started to hear a very dull and reverberating noise. At first, I thought my partner was using our suction device to clear the guy's airway for the intubation, but I soon realized the noise was coming from the patient.

A strong, pungent smell hit me right in the face and almost knocked me over. This guy was leaving his final mark on this world by letting out a long and disgusting death fart. While I was trying to compose myself and clear my eyes, my partner was almost turning purple trying to hold back laughter. I decided right then and there that when my time comes, if I don't go in my sleep, I want to be the nastiest code that a medic ever works. I know at least for those sorry few who work on me, that I won't be forgotten.

I just heard the music from an ice cream truck as it drove by, and that takes me back to the first time I met Michelle. It was December, and I had only been back to work a short time after being out four months with a broken wrist.

It would be so cool if I could tell you I broke my wrist in a skydiving accident or something like that. The truth is, I was drunk and slipped on my own marble floor while wearing socks. Just reading that makes me feel like an idiot. Maybe I should have gone with the skydiving story. You wouldn't have known the difference, but I told you I wouldn't lie while writing this, and I am keeping my word.

Anyway, I was back to work and I got dispatched to back up another unit on a three-year-old little girl who had been run over by an ice cream truck. This call was in the middle of the hood, and it looked as if a crowd was about ready to riot when we arrived on scene. The patient was already in the back of the first unit, so I jumped in to see how I could help.

Michelle had recently been hired and was riding with another crew during her orientation. Fortunately for her, on this day, one of the crew was my friend DQ. The charge medic was a girl who no longer works here and was a brownnoser.

Once inside, the atmosphere was pretty chaotic as all three were trying to cope with the situation.

Michelle, who I had never met before, seemed to have her shit together, and my boy DQ was calm as usual. The charge paramedic, on the other hand, was losing it. Looking at the child, I knew we were fighting an already lost battle. Her head had been run over by the truck's tire, and although still intact, felt like mush. I tried to intubate her, but it was impossible. Crushed teeth and brain filled her mouth, and I knew our efforts would be futile.

Even though my administration hates my ass because I speak my mind, a lot of my co-workers respect me, which I truly appreciate. I tried to play big brother on this call and help my peers deal with the situation.

"Guys, this little girl is dead, and there's nothing we can do to change that," I told them. "You are all doing a good job, so just try to take a deep breath and relax."

While DQ drove us to the ER, the back of the unit became more manageable, and we focused on doing the job at hand. I could tell Michelle was a little upset after the call and even though I didn't know her, I told her that DQ would be there for her if she needed to talk.

It wasn't long after that call that Michelle and I became partners. To this day she and her husband, who also works here, are two of my best friends.

A little side note. The parents of the dead child were in a house smoking crack at the time and blamed the Indian truck driver and us for her death while they screamed racist comments at us. Hopefully the welfare checks they receive every month will supply them with enough crack to help them get over their heartache. After a call like that, I guess I shouldn't complain about my hard-earned money being ripped away to help outstanding parents like them.

Maybe the left of the political spectrum are right. After busting my ass and risking my life every third day, I should just hand over my entire paycheck to these obviously deserving souls. I'll tell another one about an unfit parent, and this one upset every rescuer on scene. We responded to a drowning call at a motel swimming pool. This particular motel was known for being a haven for drug-heads and hookers. I was actually surprised that this place had a working swimming pool.

As we arrived on scene, we saw a small group gathered, and a lone man was performing CPR on a small child. The man had noticed the little boy at the bottom of the pool. He jumped in and pulled the kid out with no aid from the people who had come over after his cries for help.

Herocs can be right around the corner at any given moment, and you won't know it until a given situation presents itself. What that man did was heroic in my eyes.

Upon reaching the patient, we immediately began our care. The little boy was maybe three or four, and had no pulse. Our heart monitor showed asystole, which is a flatline. As we worked on the patient, the fire department and one of my supervisors arrived.

Water and vomit was coming out of the boy's mouth as a firefighter did chest compressions. We were doing everything we could to revive the little boy when his mother suddenly appeared on scene.

"What happened?" I heard the woman ask in a very mellow and almost distant tone.

While we continued to work on the patient, my supervisor asked if she was the mother. She said she was the child's mother, and that she and the scrawny-looking dirtbag with her, had only left the boy alone for a brief moment.

"We left him with that girl who is always hanging out by the front office," she said without any emotion. "We were only gone an hour, and I told him to stay away from the pool."

Every emergency worker on that scene was pissed, but it's what this dumb bitch said next that made me want to explode.

"Baby, where are my cigarettes?"

This woman's child was laying lifeless right in front of her, and she was asking some low-life who I'm guessing she had only just met about her smokes. She wasn't crying, yelling, or even acting remotely concerned about her son. She had left her child with a stranger so she could go blow some guy for a couple bucks, and she didn't even seem to care that her boy was dead. I don't care how hardcore a medic is or how long he's been on the job, seeing this kind of shit over and over wears you down.

How some people can feel sorry for a person like her really gets me. In our society today, she is looked at as the victim. She must have had a traumatic childhood, or somebody screwed her over at some point in time. Bullshit! These are the same excuses I mentioned earlier about career criminals. Is anyone ever going to be held accountable for their own actions anymore? I doubt it, and once again, you and I pay the tab.

The last call is a perfect example of why EMS workers are now included in hi-risk retirement. Like I said before, it's not the risk of being killed on the job, which is very possible and deep down is on everyone's mind. It's all the messed-up things we see and deal with that takes us to the brink. When you constantly see people fucking each other over, it breaks you down. As I've explained, high blood pressure, cardiac issues, and depression are common among seasoned EMS workers.

Everyone has a breaking point both mentally and physically. I've seen medics reach that point and just hang it up and walk away, while others hide their issues and somehow keep it together until retirement. We had a guy a long time ago who kept working even though he had obviously gone over the edge. He had been working in my service for a few years after coming down from a big city service up north. I remember riding with him a couple times as a student, and he appeared to know what he was doing. Even as a student, though, I could tell he was wired a little too tight.

Towards the end of his time with my service, he just began acting strange. He would freak out on simple mindless calls, or just sit down on a scene while his partner did all the work. One time he was driving a patient to a local hospital, and although he had taken hundreds of patients to this same facility before, he started driving in the opposite direction. When his partner realized this, he had already driven a couple miles in the wrong direction. His partner told him to turn around. Obviously disoriented, after arguing a while, he finally agreed and turned around.

I can't remember if he eventually got fired or left on his own, but I heard that people were trying to hide from him when he picked up his final paycheck. I don't know if that story is true or not, but the thought of people who don't give a shit about their employees hiding under their desks cracks me up. The stressful situations any emergency worker deals with can get to them over time, or any given call might be the one that causes a medic to reach the breaking point.

178 TONES

CHAPTER 26

Most of us are able to put up walls that hide our emotions and feelings, but we are only human. I told you earlier that talking to my friends is what keeps me going. There have been many times when I have felt like dropping my belt and walking away after a call. There's one call that I still think about all the time, and it was the one that would have pushed me over the edge had it not been for my friends.

I showed up on the scene of a very bad MVC. A car had slammed into the rear end of a broken down semi truck. The driver of the car had been talking on his cell phone and didn't notice the truck stopped in front of him. When we got to him, he was pinned under the truck. Blood was pouring out of his forehead and he was very combative, which in itself is a sign of a head injury.

A helicopter was called and had landed as we were still working to free him from the wreckage. This guy was morbidly obese and it was very difficult to extricate him. It took so long, in fact, that the chopper actually shut down its engine. They could not take a large combative patient inside the helicopter.

The flight crew began working with us as we pulled him out, and it was determined the patient needed to be RSI'd (Rapid Sequence Intubation). As the medications took effect, I tried to intubate but I couldn't see anything, so the flight medic gave it a try. After several attempts he got the intubation.

It's always an ego thing when a medic sees someone else successfully accomplish a skill that they were unable to perform, and intubations are the worst. In this case, however, I was just happy someone, anyone, had gotten the tube. Feeling as though my job was done as the flight crew and firefighters wheeled the patient to the helicopter, I pulled off my gloves and walked to my truck.

Suddenly, I heard a commotion and saw the patient was again combative. The sedation had worn off, and the patient awoke and ripped the tube from his throat. I quickly ran over and tried to help hold the patient down so he could be re-sedated.

Paralytics were again administered and the flight crew prepared to re-intubate. A flight crew, by the way, consists of a flight nurse and a flight medic. These nurses are usually ER nurses who undergo extensive training to deal with pre-hospital situations. The flight medics are no different than me except they receive special training in helicopter operations. Having personally survived a helicopter accident myself, while in the Army, I hold these crews in high regard.

What had begun as the fading light of late afternoon had now turned to a scene of darkness at night. The flight medic once again tried to intubate, but unlike the first time, the patient began to projectile vomit. Projectile vomiting looks just like it sounds. A long stream of vomit shot out of the patient's mouth about four feet in the air and was followed by a never-ending spew of puke. There was no way to intubate now, and the patient started to crash.

We looked in horror as the patient's heart rate began to *Brady*, or slow down. We could not suction him fast enough so it was agreed a cricothyrotomy was needed. I was the only one among that group who had performed one. As I stated earlier, this man was huge, and I had to have a firefighter push down on both sides of his neck just to feel any landmarks.

Feeling what I thought was the Adam's apple, I moved my fingers down until I felt what I believed to be the incision site. Both the flight medic and nurse concurred with me, and I made my first incision through the skin. I turned away briefly to grab the airway tube, and when I did, for whatever reason the firefighter released his pressure on the neck.

We lost pulses and the patient went into PEA or, Pulseless Electrical Activity. What this meant was, we were still seeing a heartbeat on the monitor, but felt no pulse. While CPR was initiated, I took my bare finger and put it into the incision which was now on the side of his throat. I attempted to blindly feel the cricoid membrane but couldn't. Watching this man die in front of me and feeling totally helpless, I cut through his trachea and tried to insert the tube. It wouldn't go in, and we started to bag him without any advanced airway. In a situation like this without any airway, simply bagging a patient is futile. He is obviously aspirating or inhaling massive amounts of vomit and blood into his lungs.

I told the flight crew to take off and that I would ground transport the patient to our closest hospital. This patient was not going to make it and the medevac helicopters don't generally take cardiac arrests. We loaded him in back of my unit and were preparing to leave when I noticed the flight nurse jump in.

"I got this," I told her. "You don't have to come." This would be my first and only call with this flight nurse. She was a short little thing, maybe five two, and Asian. Seeing her in the dim lights of the back of my truck, I realized how beautiful she was.

She seemed like a very headstrong individual. "We are in this together. I'm not going to just dump this on you," she said. She easily could have taken off and flown away, and I wouldn't have blamed her, but she didn't. This woman had integrity.

We wheeled the patient into the ER and the staff worked on him briefly before pronouncing him dead.

Even though I was covered in blood, the flight nurse gave me a hug and asked me if I was okay before leaving. I told her I was and watched her as she left the room.

I turned back to the patient and stood in what I can only describe as a state of shock. I had cut this man's throat and now he was dead. My supervisor on this night was a guy I had known a long time, and I have always respected him. He had been in the military and honestly cared about his people. He asked me if I was all right as I stood there covered in blood. It seemed as though he was talking to me through a tunnel. Every word sounded muffled. He noticed my blood-covered arms and grabbed them to see if I had been injured.

Seeing that I was all right physically, he pulled me aside to see if I still had my shit together. "I think I just killed a man," I said without any emotion.

Looking into my eyes, I think he could tell that I was fucked up. "Go home, man. I'll get on the truck for you," he said.

Most of the supervisors I've had over the years wouldn't say something like that, but he had integrity. I told him that I needed to finish the shift and that going home to an empty house would only make it worse. Several co-workers were at the hospital when we came in and came over to check on me as I sat outside smoking a cigarette on the curb. I love these people. I can't say that enough.

Before I go any further I must tell you this. A month or so after this call, the flight nurse who rode to the hospital with me was killed when her helicopter hit a pole and crashed. What a tragic end to the life of a caring and beautiful person! In her obituary I learned that she was also a flight nurse in the Air National Guard and had served in Desert Storm. I knew then where she had gotten her integrity. God bless her.

I finished my shift and was still in a daze of disbelief as I drove home. It was a Sunday morning and hardly any traffic was on the road. In the distance I saw an ambulance pull up to an intersection, and as I got closer, I noticed a fire truck and cop car. With nothing else to do, I pulled over and walked up to the scene.

A man had been hit by a car, and as I approached, my brother and sister working on him looked up at me in confusion. "What are you doing here?" they asked.

"Just passing by," I replied.

I must have been a sight. I still had dried blood on me from the night before, and I asked if I could help. They said they could use all the help they could get so I got down and intubated the patient.

I was back in my car and continuing my drive home when it dawned on me what had just happened. An hour or so after I got home, I got a call from another one of my supervisors. At first I thought he was calling to see if I was all right, considering what had happened the night before and all, but that wasn't the case.

"You need to put in an overtime voucher for that call you stopped at," he told me. That way the county couldn't be sued because I was technically off duty when I stopped to help. The fact that I had helped save the guy didn't seem to matter.

I was now off for a couple shifts on vacation and that wasn't a good thing. I completely shut down. My friends called and came by and knocked on the door, but I wouldn't answer. I spent three days isolated in my house and drank like I never had before. It was like a movie scene playing over and over again in my head. I'm holding the scalpel, cutting this guy's throat and blood is spraying all over me. I felt like Jack the Ripper and it was destroying me. I was convinced that I had killed this man.

Ask anyone who has been a soldier or marine, and they will tell you about being trained to use violence to defend their buddies, themselves, or to complete a mission. Deep down inside, we pray we'll never need that training, but we are prepared to use it all the same.

When I left the Army, I was thankful that I never had to experience hand-to-hand combat, even though I was kind of jealous of those who had. I guess that's just a macho thing. My Uncle Bill was awarded Silver and Bronze Stars in World War II for killing the enemy in close combat and it still haunts him. In the long run, I thought I got off easy until that last call.

Knife skills are something soldiers are trained in. If your weapon fails, you must be prepared to go for your bayonet, and you accept that. The fact that a man died after I had cut his throat in a failed medical procedure trying to save his life was something I couldn't accept.

Maybe I shouldn't have gone back over to the patient after I took my gloves off. I mean, after all, he was the flight crew's responsibility at that point. Maybe I shouldn't have said that I had done a couple cric's or that it appeared to be our last option. Maybe I should have just kept my fucking mouth shut. Maybes, *coulda's*, *shoulda's*, and *woulda's* didn't matter anymore. The guy was dead and I was covered in blood, if only in my mind at this point.

For three days I didn't sleep, barely ate, and didn't shower. I smelled and looked like ass, while playing my old records repeatedly on the stereo. I said I wouldn't lie while writing this, so this is my confession regarding my weakest moment. At some point during my self-sentenced confinement, I contemplated putting a gun to my head. Even though I was in a drunken stupor, I remember crying and shaking uncontrollably as I briefly considered suicide. What had I done? I wasn't a soldier anymore, and I hadn't cut an enemy's throat in combat. I was supposed to help the guy, and I had failed miserably. Fortunately, at least for me, I passed out.

When I awoke the next morning, I was on the floor of my bedroom with the sound of an old record skipping. *What the fuck?* I thought to myself.

I loved myself too much to have even contemplated suicide, and Lord knows I'm allergic to pain. That would have devastated my mother, family, and friends. Hadn't I learned anything from my girl's suicide? At some point in time, I turned my phone back on and shortly afterward, I got a call from a co-worker. He asked how I was doing and said that some of my friends were going to have the cops bust into my place if I hadn't answered the phone when I did.

I told him that I was okay and that I had just needed some space. I had known the guy for about a year and he was a good man. We weren't close or anything and I don't think we had ever even had a beer together, but I guess he had picked up on a conversation between my closer friends about my situation.

I'm not sure why, but he then got in contact with the medical examiner's office, where they explained what had happened to me. These days, with all the privacy laws, they wouldn't have told him *anything*. At that time, however, they gave him the MD's findings.

He told me that the autopsy showed massive brain trauma, and that the patient wouldn't have survived even if he didn't pull the tube. I felt like a death row inmate who was given a last-minute reprieve. Even though I knew in my heart that I hadn't killed the man, I had let my own emotions and imagination get the best of me. Emotions and imagination are something every human has, regardless of upbringing or physical and financial standing. We all have them, and they can be considered a weakness or strength. In my case they were both weaknesses, but as is human nature, I was able to turn them into strengths.

I returned to work more motivated than ever. I had been to the depths of my own personal hell and had come out stronger than ever. With all the turmoil that besieges every emergency worker, I was quickly able to forget my own bullshit and deal with the job at hand. I had friends going through divorces, custody battles, and a hell of a lot more serious situations than my own.

So what if a patient dies? As long as I know I did my best, and followed my protocols, why the hell should I care? Would any of the people I try to help care at all about me or my family's well-being? The answer is *no*, and that's the way it should be. You and your loved ones shouldn't have to worry about me and mine. That's why we're here. We do what we do, so that you and yours can live your lives in peace, even though it goes against much of what I've been preaching.

Chapter 27

Man, that's another group that drives me crazy. I'm not a preacher, and I can't stand some of the people who call themselves that. Too many preachers or evangelists, if you will, are full of shit in my eyes. I'm referring to *some*—not all of them, of course.

I have said several times that I believe in God and an afterlife, and I wasn't joking. I am not the sharpest tool in the shed by any means, which by now, after reading this far, you have already figured out. I am not stupid or ignorant, however, and I can comprehend most things.

A person has the right to believe in any religion he wants. I don't care if it's the Christian God, Allah, Buddha, or a tuna sandwich. Believe what you want to believe, it's your life. All I ask is that you don't try to force your interpretations of religion on me. I'll believe in what I want to believe, and that's that.

All around the world there are people who stand in front of crowds reading a book. It might be the Bible, the Quran, or any number of religious scriptures, and after reading the book, they put their own spin on it. Seriously, I can read and I don't want to hear their interpretations.

A book might say, "...and God..." Allah or whoever said, "... plant potatoes." The next thing you know some cleric is saying that "plant potatoes" means "bomb a nursery school." Read whatever book you choose, and take from it what you need, so long as your needs don't include *blowing shit up*. Just remember that not one of the religious figures speaking wrote what you are reading.

Holy shit! I just got religious on you, and I'm the least religious person I know. Sorry.

As I was saying before I rudely interrupted myself, the general population shouldn't be concerned with the EMS worker's personal life. Before I got into this line of work, I never thought about paramedics or EMT's. I'm even talking about before I was a soldier. I think I was like everyone else. Calling 911 meant getting a fire truck, and I was comfortable with that. I never thought or even imagined that the ambulance crews were so highly skilled and available 24/7. As I said, you should not have to concern yourselves with our personal lives—but, you should respect our abilities and commitment.

The public should rest easy knowing that when they are in need and call for help, we'll be there. They should also realize that we are there to help them and not take any bullshit.

The term *public servant* is outdated. I am not a servant for anyone. People like me are medical professionals. We have undergone extensive training to help you, to save you. Calling us servants is an insult. We have to pay the same taxes as everyone else.

Just remember that—*no matter where you go, there you are*. I'm not sure where I heard that saying, but I like it. To me it says that you should try to live life to its fullest, regardless of where you find yourself.

When I started this book, writing *was* and still *is* new to me. I've had no real literary education, but have been learning as I go. What I have learned over these last several thousand words is that anyone can express himself if he just chooses to commit to writing whatever is on his mind.

I have always loved to read but I never realized how cathartic it is to write. A person can truly just let it go and express anything he wants, and it is an awesome feeling. Simply putting my words down has been the biggest vent for me in years. I have told you, the reader, about things that I have never confessed to anyone, and it feels like a weight has been lifted off my shoulders.

I know my story is too graphic for children and even some adults, but hopefully some of our society's EMS educators or even educators in general will read this, and pass along to their students how great a feeling putting pen to paper can be.

Which reminds me, teachers are also way underpaid. I just wanted to throw that in before I get back to the main subject of my story, the EMS worker.

CHAPTER 28

I have told you how most of us in the emergency medical world are underpaid. We are also, for the most part, underappreciated. Hopefully you have learned that we are not brainless ambulance drivers, and in fact, we are highly trained medical professionals.

I'm not sure, but I think this is the first time that I've mentioned the term ambulance driver while writing this book. This moniker is not only very insulting but highly degrading. Calling my brothers and sisters or me ambulance drivers is the equivalent of calling a doctor saw bones. Yes, we do respond in an ambulance, and we have undergone extensive training to drive them, but that is not our sole purpose. If you or a loved one needs help, and you only think of us as drivers, call UPS. I know for a fact that they are paid better than us.

This reminds me of the time my co-workers and I were sitting in front of our station shooting the shit. It was time for shift change and we were all hanging out. A garbage or waste management truck pulled up to pick up our trash. I had talked to this one guy before, and he joked about how cool our jobs must be because we were just sitting around. I told him that he should be thankful, and he stopped and asked why. I said, "Because we do the same job as you but your trash doesn't talk back."

After an uncomfortable silence, he smiled and walked away, shaking his head. As I previously mentioned, my job would be perfect if not for the majority of our so-called patients. Remember what I said earlier about the majority of our calls being bullshit? Those are the patients I'm referencing and not the legit ones. I don't care who you might ask in the emergency world, if they disagree with this perspective, they are lying.

Recently my partner and I were accused by some drunken lady and her husband of stealing money from them. This is something that future EMS workers should think about before entering this profession. It seems like some people want to make a profit off calling us. In my career, co-workers and I have been accused of stealing everything from money to false teeth. I mean really, who the hell would want someone else's nasty-assed false teeth?

Anyway, on this most recent call we responded to the DAV (Disabled American Veteran) hall for an intoxicated individual. Upon arrival we found a man in his early sixties sitting at the bar. This guy was so polluted drunk that he couldn't even stand.

I approached the man and asked if he was okay. "Fuck you, motherfucker!" was his reply as he tried to slap me.

I explained to him that I was called to help him and not take his shit. That's when his extremely intoxicated wife got into the act. "He's a veteran and you can't talk to him like that!" she exclaimed.

I told her that I was a veteran and a member of the VFW, and that being a vet didn't give her husband the right to be a drunken asshole.

I have had several run-ins with so-called veterans over the years, and most of them are full of shit. I have had shitbags younger than me say that they were Vietnam vets. I mean really, what were they, three years old? My cousin John was killed in that war, so these assholes really piss me off.

Anyway, back to the drunk at the bar. We had to call law enforcement to help restrain this waste of space to our stretcher. Needless to say, the guy was a jerk all the way to the hospital, and he carried it even further with the nursing staff.

Did any of us take the man's money? Absolutely not, but because we didn't bow down and take their abuse, they figured they would fuck with us. Being in the public's eye, you must get used to having a bull's eye on your back. That goes for anyone in the emergency world, be it fire, police, or EMS. Just once

I wish I had the stones to accuse some shithead of stealing from me. I think I would say they took my solid gold stethoscope and bed pan. Unfortunately, I could never stoop to that level. I have morals, which at times can be an inconvenience.

Over the years I have dealt with a lot of assholes, and if it weren't for the fact that I believe in a God, I would have messed some of them up. Some people think that they have the right to yell at us and on some occasions touch us. I don't know where that concept came from, but if you touch my partner or me, you will get a beat down. I have been swung at, yelled at, and spit on. I have been called motherfucker, asshole, racist and so many other things I can't remember, and I never let that get to me or piss me off too much.

Like I said, the one thing that does pull the pin on my grenade is when someone touches my partner or me. When that happens, things get ugly, especially if I'm working with a female. I consider the girls I work with my little sisters, and I don't know any man who wouldn't be protective of his little sisters.

I won't go into too many details, if only to protect myself, but over the years I've had to get physical, with a few deserving souls. This isn't a macho thing, but instead, a self-preservation thing. We are not given any means of self-defense and so I, at times, have taken things into my own hands. One call always comes to mind when I think of this subject.

About ten or fifteen years ago, I ran a call on some drunken white trash biker piece of shit. This jerk got shitfaced and fell into a ditch behind a bar. When we arrived, a cop was helping him out of the ditch. This dude was huge, and very drunk. Blood was trickling down his face from a laceration on the top of his head.
I explained to him that we were there to help, and that he needed stitches. After arguing with him, he finally said we could transport him, but not on a backboard. In a normal situation we place patients with head injuries on a board to reduce the chances of cervical spine injury. This guy wasn't having it, so we placed him sitting up on the stretcher.

This call happened around midnight and I rode in the back with the patient. I was working with a female partner and I didn't want her in back. Who says chivalry is dead?   So, I'm sitting behind the patient in the captain's chair, and he decides he wants a piece of me. After disconnecting the stretcher's seatbelts, he started to get up, and I tried to hold him down. Just then, he grabbed my arm. Did I mention that I don't like being touched and that this guy was huge? Well, when I say huge, I mean he was about six foot and approximately two hundred fifty pounds.

This call was before we started using laptops, and our reports were still handwritten. I kept mine in a thick metal clipboard. We used to call these clipboards snap packs, and that title got a new meaning this night.

I have never backed down from a fight, which I must admit in the past had caused me a lot of pain. This man was certainly capable of putting a serious hurt on me. "I'm gonna kick your fuckin' ass!" were the last words he said before I slammed, or should I say snapped my metal clipboard down hard on his head.

Oh shit! I thought to myself as he slumped back down on the stretcher. I had just put a hurting on this guy, and what had been a relatively small cut on his head was now a large gaping wound.

I had really hit him hard—but better him than me, right? I wish that is what I was thinking at the time, but it wasn't. I was freaked because not only had I knocked my patient out, but now he was bleeding profusely all over the place. Instead of dressing his wounds, I spent the rest of the transport cleaning all the blood and hair off my snap pack. As we arrived at the emergency room, he started to come to, and he was pissed off. By now I had cleaned up all of the incriminating evidence, and we rolled him into the emergency room.

It was kind of funny. This hulking, tattooed, white trash piece of shit was trying to accuse me of assault and battery when I had clearly defended myself. This guy had a criminal record going back to his middle school days, and he was trying to press charges against me after attacking me in my truck. It turned out that this genius had an outstanding warrant and was hauled off to jail anyway. This man should not have been on the street in the first place, considering his record. He had proven over and over that he didn't care about others. Through his actions, I could have potentially been seriously injured or lost my career, even though I was clearly defending myself.

This might make you think. Since that call, I have saved numerous lives, and there are people walking this earth today because of my actions. Actually, action is a poor choice of word. There are people alive today because of my extensive training and experience, and if this one dickbag would have had his way, I would have lost my certification. I'm not saying my peers couldn't have had the same success with these saves, but I was the charge paramedic on these calls.

Unfortunately, this great country of ours has taken a twisted view on reality, as I've detailed before. The social waste that victimizes the innocent are the ones looked upon as the victims, and some actually think that criminals and 911 abusers should be coddled. This is such an unrealistic point of view that it can only be taken by those who have never seen the reality of the streets. People who have never seen firsthand the horrors that the EMS worker sees can easily hide in their glass houses. I wish I had that luxury, but instead I choose to work in that same harsh world and try to make a difference—and yes, I've paid a price mentally and physically for it.

When you see a beautiful baby that will grow up permanently brain damaged because some asshole didn't like her crying so he shook her too hard, that will make you think. When you see another beautiful child who was raped at age twelve and had so much trauma done to her immature reproductive organs that she will never be able to have her own children—that will make you think.

My God! How I wish I could erase those images from my mind, but I can't. In a way I guess it's a good thing, because it keeps me grounded in this very real and cruel world. It also lets me be a voice for them, the true victims of our society.

You may want to turn your head or switch channels so you can avoid the harsh reality of this life. However, the truth is, whenever you see an EMS worker, you are staring straight at it. For we see and deal with it every day so you don't have to. You may not understand us, or ever even think about us, and that's okay. All I can ask is that you respect us, or at the very least accept us for who we are and what we do.

We are not mindless civil servants or ambulance drivers. We, as a whole, are your fellow man and woman who have chosen to try to make a difference. We don't want false praise or unnecessary accolades. We simply want to be acknowledged for what we are, paramedics and EMTs.

I have tried to express this through my writing, and my story is just one of thousands. I hope I have been able to accomplish what I set out to do at the beginning, which was to shine an honest light. It wasn't pretty, I know, but it was like I promised, true. I am a very opinionated person for which I won't apologize. Considering all I have seen and experienced in my life, I think I deserve to be.

That's one of the great things left in America, the freedom to speak your mind or in this case, write it. It is funny how there are so many people who never once wore a uniform in defense of this country, but totally take advantage of this freedom given to them. Freedom of speech—what an awesome and powerful thing!

It is not my intention to belittle those who didn't serve, because not everyone hears the call. In fact, less than one percent of our population chooses to serve. I am, however, going to slam the assholes who recite the First Amendment while bashing this country, and never once stood up to defend that right. I have seen a lot of celebrities do this over the years. Subjects like Hurricane Katrina and the wars we are in come to mind when I think about this. With Katrina you had famous people calling Bush a racist. He wasn't a racist he was an idiot with poor advisors. People from every race suffered in the aftermath. I know firsthand how devastating a hurricane can be after performing search and rescue following Hurricane Charley.

As for the war on terror, when I see entertainers complain about stuff like water boarding prisoners it blows my mind. This only motivates the people who hate our country and want to kill us. I've yet to see any complain about our prisoners who have been executed.

I really wish people with access to the media would think before they speak.

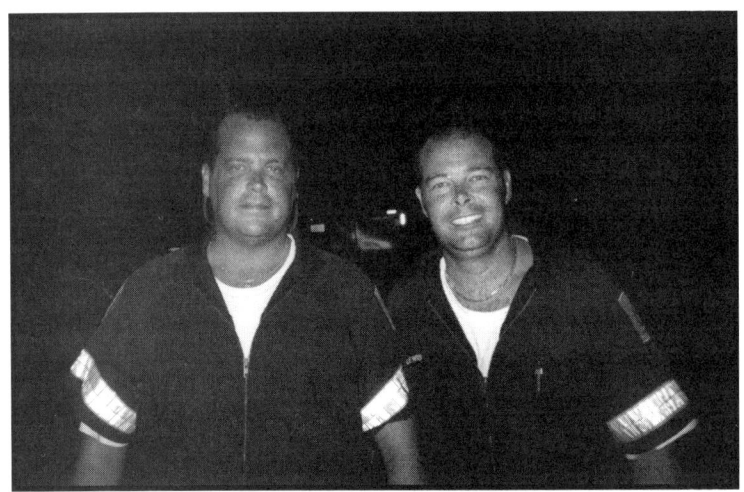
Me and my friend Jay after 30 straight hours of search and rescue following Hurricane Charley.

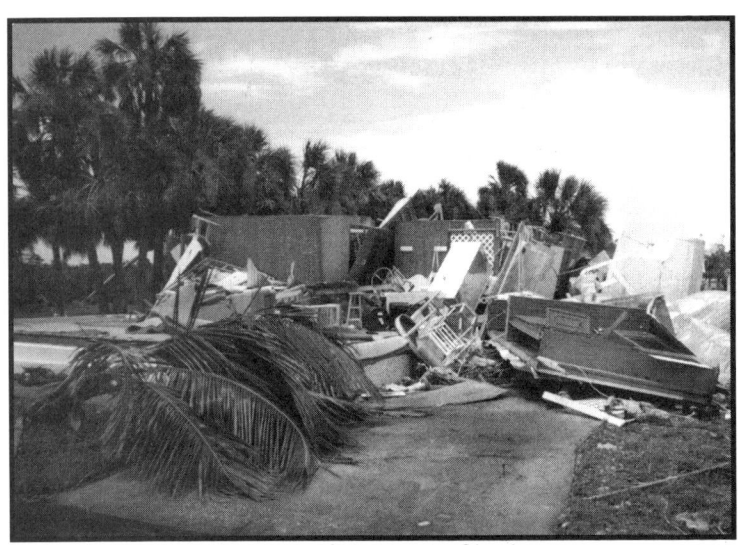
Aftermath of Hurricane Charley.

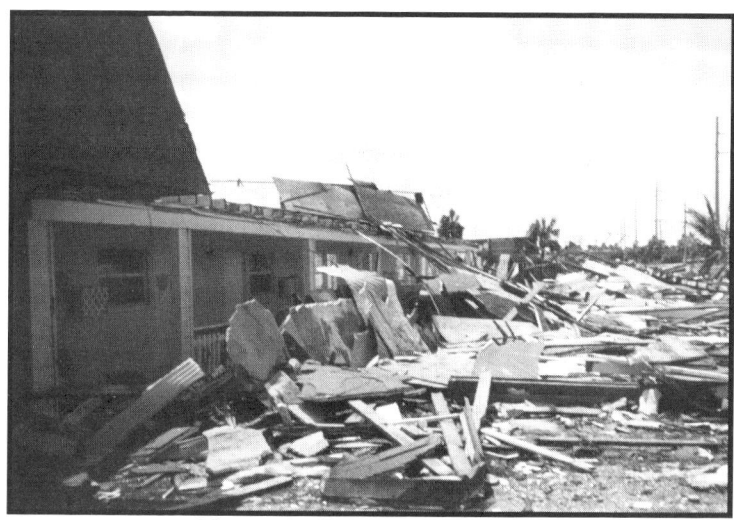

Aftermath of Hurricane Charley.

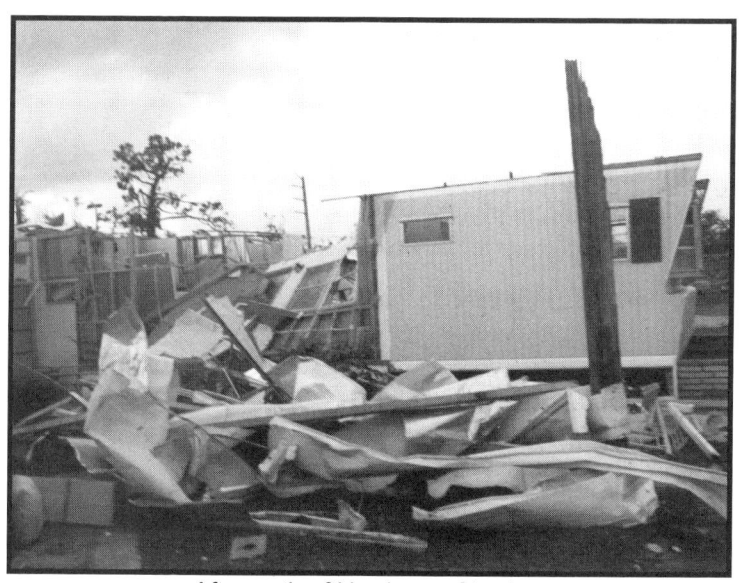

Aftermath of Hurricane Charley.

204 TONES

Chapter 29

Working in the emergency field also means not knowing when you'll see your family, friends, pets, or even your house again. I'm not talking about being injured or killed. I'm talking about being forced to work against your will.

In my service this is called *being held over* or *drafted*. Mine is not the only emergency service that does this. I'm sure every EMS service or fire department has a similar policy. *Holdover* means that there are not enough personnel to man the trucks so we can be forced to stay for an additional 24 hours.

In my service, holdover is almost a daily event. It's one thing to be held for a catastrophic emergency like a hurricane, for which I have been several times. But to be drafted for what should be a routine workday is something else.

Can you imagine completing a long workday, and just as you were preparing to go home, being told you have to stay for another shift? How could you plan anything for off days? Believe me, it's hard.

I work a lot of voluntary overtime shifts just to make up for an already below average wage. Yes, I know this country is in a financial crisis and that most of us are hurting. However, our pay sucked even during the real estate boom before the recent blunder by our trusted politicians.

I have been held over several times during my career and some of those were after I'd already worked back-to-back double shifts. Talk about burn out. I can understand the need to keep the trucks running and I accept being held over without argument. It's the fact that nothing is done to prevent it that irks me.

I know our commissioners and directors don't have to worry about forced labor, and by definition, that's exactly what it is. Hell, some of them already have successful businesses on the side or are already retired with sweet pensions, and our taxes still give them fat cash and benefits. What a waste of money! If they care so much about our community, they should work for half of what they're paid. Their benefits and perks alone could make up for the rest. Being a taxpaying homeowner myself, I have no problem saying that.

It's not me or my brothers' and sisters' fault that the department has a high turnover rate, or that people get fed up with the non-proactive work environment and low pay—and quit. Yet again, we are the ones who bear the burden. I know people who've missed flights because they were held over on the first day of vacation. I know single parents who had to jump through hoops at the last minute just to find somebody to watch their children for another 24 hours.

This is not whining, folks. This is simply someone trying to bring light to a subject long ignored. If the unfair things I've mentioned and will mention involved a single sex or race, people would be outraged and crying for justice. So, if it helps, imagine for a moment that EMS workers are green with tails. Just for the record, I don't whine—I bitch. There is a difference.

Unfortunately, this is another negative factor that people should contemplate before committing to a career in emergency medicine. For EMS, fire, and police, in my home state of Florida, it looks like things might be getting worse. Some of the higher politicians in my state are trying to get rid of the high risk retirement to save some of the taxpayers' money. Not only has it been proven that we are at higher risk for health issues, but now they want us to work past our projected life expectancy. I guess in a way, it will save money because we won't be able to use our pension. We'll be dead before we qualify.

I remember one of these politicians campaign commercials. It showed his elderly mother talking about how great her son was. It was typical cheesy political crap. I wonder now how his mom would feel about him if she fell and couldn't get up and nobody came to her aid because every emergency worker quit. That's a grim scenario and I hope it never comes true, but if his vision comes to fruition, why would anyone want to do this job?

There's an old saying in the emergency world, "If you go into this field to make money, you've chosen the wrong career." None of us got into this for the money, but is hoping to make a decent living and enjoying a much deserved retirement too much to ask? It's almost as if some think we should just be happy to help everyone else and not care about ourselves or loved ones. I could be wrong but that just doesn't make any sense to me.

In my county there are taxes for the Sheriff's Department and the individual fire departments. EMS, on the other hand, is grouped in with the rest of the other departments like Public Works and we have to share those revenues in addition to the small amount collected from medicare and health insurance. To me, this is the most obvious of examples of the lack of support of EMS. Again, all I can say is *remember Arby's*. For years I've seen brand new police cars with stickers on the windows parked around our station. They are never even started, let alone moved. The tax money wasted on those cars could have been used for vehicles that actually serve a purpose, like an ambulance.

Even better, the money could have been used to bring our pay to a decent wage. Now, I'm not a politician and we know how wise and caring they are.

But if they did things to keep EMS employees from quitting, they would, in the long run, be saving money. They would not have to pay overtime to cover shifts or hold over people to keep the trucks running. This would also cut down on sick time and workers comp because people wouldn't get burned out or worn down. I think that sounds logical, doesn't it?

I can't blame the local politicians for spending and taxing in the wrong places because they are just continuing what our predecessors started and they're mirroring what our national governments does. We keep giving money to so-called needy countries even though ours is severely in debt. Why are we feeding starving kids in foreign nations that wouldn't lift a finger to help our kids? I can't tell you how many children suffering malnutrition in my own community go unnoticed. Our taxes are helping everyone else but us. Enough is enough already!

There is talk in our town about possibly pulling one of our units off the road due to the budget cuts. We barely have enough trucks as it is! Our adjoining county to the south runs approximately the same amount of rescue calls as we do with almost twice as many ambulances—and we are contemplating pulling one. Someone obviously doesn't know how to manage a budget. I'm sure that that, too, will be blamed on the EMS personnel.

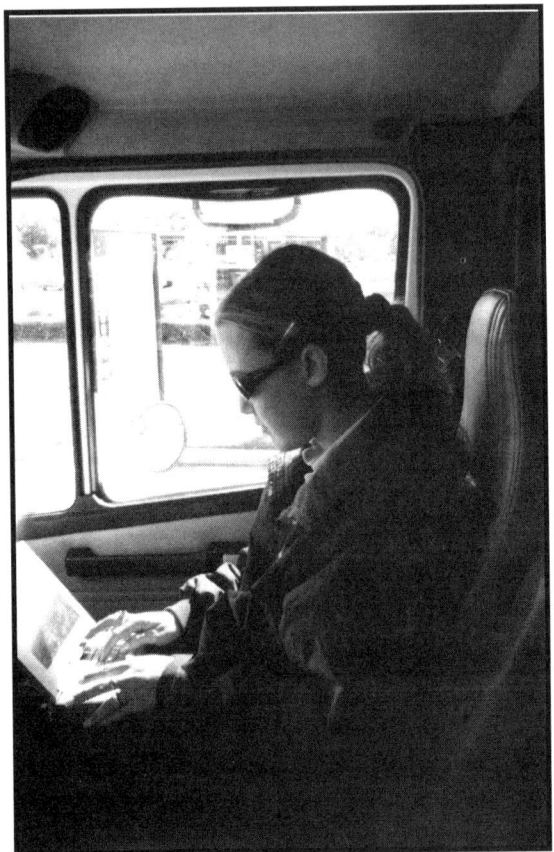

My EMS sister Jenny, typing a patient care report. She's a true friend and awesome medic.

We have a very wealthy community in the eastern part of our county where two of our units are stationed. These trucks are stationed a relatively short distance apart and run some of the fewest calls because of the location. Instead of taking a truck off the road, we should be moving one of those units in town where the majority of calls are. That will never happen, of course, because out east is where the money is. The wealthy shouldn't have to suffer because of the common people, right?

Speaking of the financially privileged, I would rather run on a drunken dirtbag than a rich asshole. At least the dirtbag can plead ignorance. The more fortunate can, on the other hand, feel free to be self-absorbed jerks. How some people can actually feel like the world owes them for being well-off is something I'll never understand. Those of us who work hard and weren't handed things on a silver platter don't owe anyone a damn thing.

All right, that was another lengthy rant about the injustices in our world. Once again, I should offer an apology for it, but I don't think I will this time. Admit it, this is something that crosses most of our minds from time to time, and it felt good for someone else to actually bring it up. Didn't it?

Like I said at the beginning, I am going to talk about many things, with some not necessarily involving EMS, but they do interact or affect EMS as a whole. Taxes, politics, and religion affect us all, so hopefully these common bonds will better help nonemergency affiliated people understand us.

Another one of my closest friends is a girl named Jenny. Like Michelle, Jackie, and Angie, she's like a little sister to me. We have never run any memorable calls together, but she has proven to be one of my best friends.

I have watched her mature as a medic since she first started here about six years ago, and I can say without any hesitation that she is one of the best medics in our service. It's funny that whenever she questions herself about a call, she will ask me for advice. More often than not, it turns out she did a better job than I would have.

Jenny was one of the few people who would go with me to visit James when he was dying. When I broke my wrist, she'd drive me to see him. She took his death very hard just like I did. I told her I would find a way to mention her in my book and I can think of no better reason than her loyal friendship and love for James. For those of us who do stick it out in this place, a few strong friendships do evolve.

There, I started this chapter off on a negative note but ended on a positive. I knew I had that in me.

CHAPTER 30

Oh well, such is life, and I am but a lowly medic telling a story. I hope my personal story has provided you some enlightenment, and no, I'm not talking about my own personal views on politics and religion. That's another cool thing about this country. You can believe or support either of those freely, without being shot.

I'm hoping that you have picked up on some of the more important and pertinent things I've mentioned—the things that just might keep you and your loved ones safe in the future. So many things go on in this busy and technologically-advanced and impersonal world that we forget the simple things. I am guilty of this too, and I openly confess to my shortcomings in this area.

I dog people all the time for yakking on cell phones while behind the wheel, and I will plead no contest to be an offender myself. I have answered a lot of calls on my cell while driving when I should have let them go to voice mail. I can say in my own defense, however, that I have never called or sent a text while driving, but that doesn't let me off the hook. A distraction is what it is, and nothing is too important that one can't pull over at the next safe spot to take a call. Yes, I will follow that simple rule from now on.

Let's call, "NOT talking on cell phones or texting while driving," number one. Number two, for the love of God, please wear a seat belt. I mean, really, how many lazy folks' brains do I have to see splattered across the road before people get the fucking point?

Most of my girlfriends are going to get pissed for me writing the following, but I write it out of love. "The seat belt hurts my boobs!" is the most common excuse I hear from women, and that's even coming from my EMS sisters. What the hell? I mean, would you rather have a brief cleavage discomfort or get shot through a windshield at high speed? It's your choice. If it were me personally, I'd go with bruised boobs over a painful death, but that's just me.

Three, learn CPR. Well, that's obviously a no-brainer. I can tell you from personal experience that bystander CPR does save lives. This is one thing that movies and TV shows have gotten right. Doing *something*, even if you're not a medical professional, is better than doing nothing. That is, unless you just don't give a shit. In that case, stay the hell out of my way because I do. CPR is such an easy thing to learn. Trust me, in the long run learning it will pay off for you sometime. Who knows, you might be a hero in somebody's eyes someday.

Four, be an organ donor. Even if you're rich and covered in makeup, you can't take it with you. If you have to, be vain and tell yourself that you will live on in some other beautiful person, because you will. Not only will you be helping others, you will be a real hero. In the next life you'll be thankful.

Who says that there is an afterlife, you ask? I don't know, the concept has been around longer than me, and it helps me continue doing my job if I think there is one. Besides, like I said before, if there *isn't*, we won't know it anyway.

Five, suicide is not the answer, unless you are suffering from a terminal and painful illness. In that case I don't think anyone has the right to blame you, even God. The only other reason I would condone suicide is if you're, say, a child molester about to get busted. If that's the case, please, feel free to blow your brains out. For all others, please realize that suicide is a permanent solution to a temporary problem. I didn't coin that last statement, but it is very true. Please seek help. You may not think so, but people do care, and your life is worth living. Trust me, the pain suicide causes loved ones and friends will only tarnish your memory and hurt the very people you love.

Six, please think before you call 911. Does the reason you're calling 911 really warrant an ambulance or do you just need a good band-aid?

In closing, let me just say this. Please rest easy with the thought that when you call 911, we will be there for you. Day or night we will come to your aid and bust our asses trying to save you. We won't prejudge or blame you, and we will sacrifice ourselves for you. All we ask is for a little respect for what we do and who we are, because as you've just read, you don't know the things that we have seen.

Is your emergency important to us? Of course it is. All true emergencies are important, and you and your loved ones are important. This is, however, a double-edged sword. Call us when you truly need us and not for selfish, meaningless bullshit reasons. When we arrive, remember who we are. We are not brainless, lower-class idiots who will accept abuse. We are highly-skilled medical professionals willing to put ourselves into difficult situations to help you and to save you. Show us our deserved respect, and you or your loved ones will get that extra mile. And who knows? When you open your door, that paramedic standing at the threshold just might be me.